THE ULTIMATE GUIDE TO

NATURAL
PAIN RELIEF

Keith Scott-Mumby MD, MB ChB, HMD, PhD

Illustrations by Oliver Scott-Mumby
www.CitizenMoose.com

The Ultimate Guide to Natural Pain Relief
By Keith Scott-Mumby MD, MB ChB, HMD, PhD

Copyright © 2014 ALL RIGHTS RESERVED

Disclaimer

ISBN: 978-0-9884196-4-3

Published by Mother Whale Inc. PO Box 371225, Las Vegas, NV, 89137

Printed in the United States of America

CONTENTS

.

INTRODUCTION

Understanding Pain

Pain isn't wholly a negative thing. It doesn't feel good but it has a useful purpose. Pain is basically telling you something is wrong and you need to take action. Typically, fixing the problem fixes the pain. Of course, this is a very simplistic view of pain but it all starts from this premise.

It is curious that people have found that the boundary between pain and pleasure is very tenuous and at times it may even disappear. Certain sexual activity can render pain a bitter-sweet stimulus and rough handling, or the deeper level of spanking and so-called sado-masochism, for many individuals, is a source of gratification, however unlikely to those who do not share the interest.

On similar lines, it is simple to observe, though rarely remarked and discussed, that the movements and facial expression of an individual at the moment of orgasm are virtually identical to someone in great pain. Even the sounds uttered are indistinguishable from those emitted in agony.

If the dividing line between pain and pleasure is so slight then it may be possible, in the light of fuller knowledge, to push a suffering patient back over the threshold in the more favorable direction, without ignoring the disease process that has heralded itself.

That's what we are going to investigate.

Blockage

Hippocrates gave us the term *ponos* and from it comes our word pain. He meant the body's fight back. Without it, there is no disease process but we would quickly die. The ensuing turmoil may be unpleasant but it is a necessary part of the limiting process.

We must not lose sight of this important fact, which is constantly being reinvented. The famous surgeon-anatomist John Hunter observed almost two centuries ago: "There is a circumstance attending accidental injury which does not belong to disease - namely, that the injury done has in all cases a tendency to produce the disposition and the means of cure."

If you block symptoms, you block the natural defenses, too. This can limit the body's own reckoning with the disease process: it fails to expel the disease properly. Long-term problems then become likely and modern medicine is nothing if not about chronic disease and its management. Have we created our own lingering pathology by constantly damping down symptoms and so thwarting the full healing process?

The alternative healer's' view of pain is that it denotes blocked energy. Where natural life force is held back or stopped, then build-ups can occur and sooner or later these announce themselves as pain. A simple example would be a gallstone or kidney stone; these impact in their respective drainage ducts, obstructing all other flow, and anyone who has experienced the resultant colic will know that it is severe pain indeed, until the blockage is relieved.

Psychosomatic Is Still Pain!

It is fashionable, though to me useless, to divide pain into what is supposed to be real pain and what is "in the mind." The total folly of this view is that *all pain is in the mind*. Think about this! Pain is just a perception, an interpretation of signals. True, there are reflex responses to stimuli that are so fast that the mind could not possibly have time to be involved, at least in the simple neurological model.

But the action (say, withdrawing a hand from a hot surface) is done without any feeling of discomfort whatever. Done quickly enough, there may be no sensation of pain at all, though a fraction of a second longer could have resulted in very unpleasant sensations and the beginning of tissue damage.

The fact is that "pain", as such, is centrally organized and perceived. That being so, why bother to distinguish between peripheral pain and that which is felt centrally but without any (apparent) visceral or somatic cause?

It is particularly unworthy of doctors to show a pejorative attitude towards the latter, while supposing the former is the only one in need of help and relief. At the end of the day, pain is pain. If the patient has it, he or she is distressed. If it is supposedly created in the mind (psychosomatic), then this must be for some purpose and it is the physician's job, no less than for "real" pain, to find the cause and bring relief from suffering.

What is wrong with a patient anyway, that he or she wants to fake something as awful as pain to get attention?

I have a similar theory about mental pain and distress; in a way it comes about through blocking communication and thus prevents healing with words. Instead of the difficulty being solved quickly and easily, it festers and builds up through time, until there is a day of undeniable pain (divorce, bereavement, redundancy, etc.)

Definition

What focuses our attention is the very unpleasant character of pain. That may have grown out of an evolutionary trend: animals that tend to pass over moderate pain may die out quickly because they are not protecting themselves. Those creatures that feel pain more unpleasantly, respond to its demands and so survive better or longer. That's the theory, anyway.

Again, it's simplistic. It makes sense, but what about animals that don't seem to feel pain? Even humble species offer some clues that they experience something of the kind that we identify as pain. An octopus, for example, exhibits real pain-like reactions, whereas many even smaller creatures don't seem to have enough brain tissue to process sensations in the way we would consider "pain".

Pain is defined by the International Association for the Study of Pain as "an unpleasant sensory and emotional experience associated with actual or potential tissue damage, or described in terms of such damage." The word *emotional* is added because the fact that we don't like it is part of our perception of pain; it generates mental as well as physical feelings: fear, sad effect, or loathing.

However, for non-human animals, it is harder, if even possible, to know whether an emotional experience has occurred. Therefore, according to Wikipedia, this concept is often excluded in definitions of pain in animals, such as that provided by American zoologist Michael Zimmerman: "an aversive sensory experience caused by actual or potential injury that elicits protective motor and vegetative reactions..."

Translation: *the animal is reacting as if it encountered something negative that it didn't like and wanted to escape from.*

The standard measure of pain in humans is how a person reports that pain, for example, on a pain scale. Only the person experiencing the pain can know the pain's quality and intensity, and the degree of suffering. Non-human animals cannot report their feelings to humans in the same manner as human communication, but observation of their behavior provides a reasonable indication as to the extent of their pain.

Nociception

We call the apparatus for creating noxious signals, for the purpose of protection from damage, nociception (same root as the word *noxious*: harmful, poisonous, damaging, unpleasant).

The subjective component of pain involves conscious awareness of both the sensation (its location, intensity, quality, etc.) and the unpleasantness (the aversive, negative affect). The brain processes underlying conscious awareness of the unpleasantness (suffering) are not well understood.

Whether you have injured yourself, harbor an infection, are experiencing an inflammatory or degenerative reaction, like arthritis, or burned yourself, the pain starts with the release of a number of irritant chemicals, known as kinins and prostaglandins.

These, in turn, trigger the sensitive nerve endings (receptors), which send signals up the line, partly as an electrical impulse, partly as a chemical response. We have nerve endings for pressure, temperature, and, of course, pain. Related pain receptors can signal a variety of challenges, including extremes of temperature and the presence of toxic chemicals, such as lactic acid, which makes muscles hurt.

The actual hardware consists of a special set of nerve-conducting fibers, known to be associated exclusively with pain signals. These fibers are thin and work relatively slowly, whereas ordinary nerve fibers, such as touch and temperature sensation, are thicker and transmit signals much more quickly than pain fibers. This is of crucial importance to the functioning of the gate-control mechanism (see below).

There are other ways in which these two types of fibers differ. Pain fibers can grow back when damaged, whereas normal nerve fibers cannot, on the whole.

There is also a third type of nerve involvement, which comes about from signals travelling downwards (retro) from the brain, which will modify the response to incoming signals.

The Gate-Control Theory

One of the great discoveries in physiology in the last fifty years has been the elicitation of the pain "gating" mechanism. The recognition of its existence is credited to Ronald Melzack, at that time (1965) an Associate Professor at MIT, and Patrick Wall, a leading British neuroscientist. Melzack and Wall reasoned that only a certain amount of information can be effectively processed by the nervous system at any moment time. If there is too much information, some of it gets dumped. Pain is the type of signal most likely to get dumped.

The gating theory says that there exists a mechanism in the spinal cord that works like a garden gate and only allows a certain number of messages through at once. Any further messages will overload the system and switch off the flow or "close the gate.". Thus a similar kind of pain or injury can be felt very differently: either quite mild or really severe, depending on how wide the gate is open at the time.

It's a simple and neat mechanism and seems to fit all the facts. It relies on the fact that pain messages, travelling up the thinner fibers, arrive at the spinal cord slightly later than touch and pressure messages from the thicker nerve fibers.

This mechanism explains a common observation, which is that by massaging the injured part or squeezing it tightly, the pain is lessened. Physical pressure near the site of injury sends plenty of messages upwards and these tend to close the gate, before the pain signals get through.

TENS (transcutaneous electrical nerve stimulation) works by electrically overloading pain fibers, so they can no longer fire properly (section 1).

Signals travelling downwards can also block the gate, which is why, when you are concentrating on a task really intently, you tend not to feel pain much. The brain is sending messages outwards, to the periphery, which block incoming signals. That's why people may not notice they have been injured right away. The mind is occupied by something more important (at least for the moment).

Three Dimensions of Pain Theory

The gating theory is not the last word in pain science.

That same Robert Melzack and another researcher, Kenneth Casey at McGill University, published a another significant paper in 1968 describing pain in terms of its three dimensions: "sensory-discriminative" (sense of the intensity, location, quality and duration of the pain); "affective-motivational" (unpleasantness and urge to escape the unpleasantness); and "cognitive-evaluative" (cognitions such as appraisal, cultural values, distraction and hypnotic suggestion).

In more everyday terms, these three dimensions are:
  * Quality, intensity and location of the pain (how much?)
  * How unpleasant it feels (how bad?)
  * The mind's attitude and how it processes the pain (so what?)

[Melzack R, Casey KL. Sensory, motivational and central control determinants of chronic pain: A new conceptual model. In: Kenshalo DR, ed. *The skin senses: Proceedings of the first International Symposium on the Skin Senses, held at the Florida State University in Tallahassee, Florida.* Springfield, IL: Thomas; 1968: 432.]

The pair theorized that pain intensity and quality are not simply determined by the magnitude of the painful stimulus, but "higher" cognitive activities can influence perceived intensity and unpleasantness.

That's another way of saying what I just said: intense mental engagement can render one temporarily numb to pain sensation. But it's also saying we can do it purposefully; lose the pain by conquering it with the mind. Even placebos can work in this way.

Thus, excitement in games or war appears to block the first dimension of pain, while suggestion and placebos may modulate the second dimension, without changing the first dimension much.

OK, so far?

By God, Sir, I've Lost My Leg!

The paper ends with a call to action: "Pain can be treated not only by trying to cut down the sensory input by anesthetic block, surgical intervention and the like, but also by influencing the motivational-affective and cognitive factors as well."

Just how well that can work is illustrated by a famous anecdote from the Battle of Waterloo. Lord Uxbridge was sitting on a horse, next to The Duke Of Wellington, when his right leg was taken off by a cannonball. He said calmly, "By God, sir, I've lost my leg!", to which Wellington looked down and replied, "By God, sir, so you have!"

The engagement in such a ferocious battle was so intense, that pain wasn't felt right away. Even during the clean-up surgery afterwards (anesthetics were still in the future, of course), Uxbridge smiled and said, "I have had a pretty long run. I have been a beau these forty-seven years, and it would not be fair to cut the young men out any longer."

Wellington was known as "The Iron Duke" but I think Uxbridge was pretty sanguine too. Tough as nails!

The point is that the brain and our mind experience can shut out pain completely, even without an anesthetic. The degree of stimulation needs to be very high indeed: at the life-and-death level.

The Chemical Basis of Pain

Pain is a complicated process that involves an intricate interplay among a number of important chemicals found naturally in the brain and spinal cord. There are also inflammatory signals within the tissues.

In general, neurotransmitters transmit nerve impulses from one cell to another. There are many different neurotransmitters in the human body; some are involved in pain and act in various combinations to produce painful sensations in the body. Some chemicals govern mild pain sensations; others control intense or severe pain.

One brain chemical of special interest to neuroscientists is glutamate. During experiments, mice with blocked glutamate receptors show a reduction in their responses to pain. Other important receptors in pain transmission are opiate-like receptors. Morphine and other opioid drugs work by locking on to these opioid receptors, switching on pain-inhibiting pathways or circuits, and thereby blocking pain (see page 16).

Receptors in the skin that responds to painful stimuli are called nociceptors. Nociceptors are thin nerve fibers in the skin, muscle, and other body tissues that, when stimulated, carry pain signals to the spinal cord and brain. Normally, nociceptors only respond to a strong stimulus, such as a pinch. However, when tissues become injured or inflamed, as with a sunburn or infection, they release chemicals that make nociceptors much more sensitive and cause them to transmit pain signals in response to even gentle stimuli such as breeze or a caress.

The most important chemicals involved with stimulating pain receptors are of various types, notably kinins, prostaglandins, and substance P. The discovery of substance P was reported in 1931, but its role then was a mystery. Now, after almost 70 years of investigation, substance P is perhaps the best understood neuropeptide transmitter. It appears to modulate nociception in the spinal cord.

Bradykinin is one of the main kinins known and it had been discovered by the time I was at medical school in the 1960s. Kinins are responsible for the generation of pain, swelling, and the cellular damage associated with inflammatory joint disease.

Not only that, but they release a second wave of inflammatory chemicals, called the cytokines. You may even have come across these names, if you are an avid reader; they include interleukin-1, tumor necrosis factor, interleukin-8, prostaglandins, and leukotrienes.

Prostaglandins are known to dramatically potentiate the pain-inducing effects of kinins.

There are two series of prostaglandins, series 1 and 2 (PGE-1 and PGE-2). In simple terms, the series 1 prostaglandins are helpful and quench inflammation, the series 2 prostaglandins cause inflammation. Also, PGE-1 comes from the omega-3 series of fatty acids, whereas PGE-2 comes from omega-6s. We do need both for proper functioning—but we DON'T need inflammation!

Other less obvious chemicals may come into play as well; for example, lactic acid build-up in muscles—the result of anaerobic exercise over a period of more than a few minutes—will produce significant pain (but lactic acid is no longer thought to be the cause of soreness and stiffness over subsequent hours and days).

Really, that's enough here. We don't need to go deeper.

Endorphins and Enkephalins

Just as we have painful substances to make pain sensations work, we also have natural onboard painkillers to fend off pain.

Endorphins and enkephalins are the body's natural painkillers. There is a third group of substances, the dynorphins, which I shall not mention again. When a person is injured, pain impulses travel up the spinal cord to the brain. The brain then releases endorphins and enkephalins. Enkephalins block pain signals in the spinal cord. Endorphins are thought to block pain principally at the brain stem.

Endorphins ("endogenous morphine") are natural opiates that function as neurotransmitters. They are produced by the pituitary gland and the hypothalamus in vertebrates during exercise, excitement, pain, consumption of spicy food, love, and orgasm, and they resemble the opiates in their abilities to produce analgesia and a feeling of well-being.

Today, the word "endorphin" is often used generically to describe three groups of opiate-type painkillers, which include enkephalins (methionine and leucine), endorphins (alpha, beta, gamma, and delta), and a growing number of synthetic (artificial) compounds.

These neurotransmitters are released by the brain and central nervous system when the brain perceives pain. The goal of pain suppression is to allow the body to cope with pain while remaining focused, rather than permitting the perception of pain to flood the system and cause panic, distress, or confusion.

In addition to dulling the sensation of pain, typically in the short term, endorphins also change the way in which people perceive pain. This may be important, because people can still be panicked or upset even when their pain is dulled, a problem that commonly occurs when people are given synthetic painkillers, which allay pain without addressing underlying emotions.

Since these neurotransmitters clearly influence perception, they play a role in memory formation and mood. They can also influence appetite and the functioning of the digestive system. All of these physical and emotional changes can be beneficial for someone experiencing pain, making the release of endorphins and enkephalins an important part of the body's response to pain and injury.

Women Experience Pain Differently Than Men

It is generally accepted that women experience pain differently than men and that their threshold for pain is less. However, you will be very surprised to learn that almost all pain research has been carried out on men and male animals, so this supposition may not be all that valid.

The argument goes that women are not good research subjects, because their lives are complicated by the menses. This is not a good line to take: given that pain is mainly a female problem, research that excludes females is incomplete at best and invalid at worst.

What is not arguable is that women complain more of pain, both in frequency and what is perceived as pain. I used to notice in my clinic that women outnumbered men about 8 to 1 and I used to remark flippantly that it's either because women whine more or women are more responsible with their health. This is the same proposition in regard to pain.

I think it is true that women do respond more to their body signals. It partly a social thing (women talk to women in ways that men would scarcely understand) and partly because women don't let things pass without taking action.

The only other thing to enter into the discussion is that testosterone does seem to blunt pain, whereas estrogen may intensify pain or blunt it. In fact it's been theorized that changing estrogen levels is really what sensitizes a woman to pain, not the actual amount of the hormone.

The effect of hormones is clearly seen in the fact that, before puberty, boys and girls respond to pain in just about the same degree. After puberty, certain types of pain are more common in girls, and even if the incidence is the same, reported pain severity is more intense in girls than boys, especially for headaches and abdominal pain. This pattern persists through adulthood; for instance, the lifetime prevalence for migraines is 18% for women and 6% for men.

One thing is clear: In this culture, women are often encouraged to express pain, and men to hide it. But this doesn't mean that friends, relatives — and doctors — react sympathetically to women's expression of pain. There is certainly a gender bias.

Alternative Methods of Pain Control

This book is an important manual on pain control because it does not dwell on all the usual solutions, meaning painkillers and other drugs. Yes, of course, there is a section on analgesics and orthodox pain control clinics, mainly for completeness. But I espouse a completely different approach from the conventional one.

Instead of simply the masking of discomfort, I believe in attempting to understand and heal the problem that causes the body to transmit pain signals.

There is always a cause. The body does not create pain purely spitefully, just to hurt the person. It is a signal of a problem, as I said at the start of this introduction. It is an imperative that is demanding a solution be found to the problem. The body rewards us immediately by the fact that the pain just goes away.

In a sense, despite the title of the book, we should not be treating the pain, but solving the causes of pain.

Any other approach smacks of folly and is unlikely to succeed in the long-term. Simply masking the symptom makes as much sense as blanking out the oil warning light on an automobile and declaring, "There, problem fixed!" We all know that, eventually, a fateful disaster will overtake the vehicle which may destroy it completely. That's not good medicine, just to cover up warning signs.

OK, let's start with pain-killing medicines…

UNDERSTANDING PAIN PRESCRIPTIONS

Pain is a very important contact point between orthodox and alternative medicine. Conventional doctors would not welcome you muscling in on cancer treatments, infectious diseases, injuries, allergies, or dermatology. But pain is something where they soften and yield: ANYTHING that can help the patient be more comfortable is tried and tolerated, no matter how bizarre (in their eyes), if it works.

The Ladder of Analgesia

We can now construct a simple four-rung ladder of analgesic use, depending on the severity of the pain.

Mild Pain
Soluble aspirin or paracetamol/acetaminophen if you are sensitive to aspirin.

Not So Mild
Aspirin with a non-steroidal anti-inflammatory drug (NSAID) such as ibuprofen.

Worse Than That
Aspirin, acetominophen/paracetamol, an NSAID such as ibuprofen, and/or acetominophen/paracetamol in a combination product with a weak opioid such as tramadol may provide greater relief than their separate use. There are combination drugs available.

Severe Pain
It partly depends if the pain condition is acute or chronic. Certain medications may work better for acute pain, others for chronic pain, and some may work equally well on both. Acute pain medication is for rapid onset of pain such as from an inflicted trauma or to treat post-operative pain. Chronic pain medication is for alleviating long-lasting, ongoing pain.

Generally speaking, when the pain is severe, doctors should switch to opiates, such as tramadol (mild) or morphine (stronger). The potential for addiction is not nearly as great as supposed (see below) and inadequate treatment of severe pain is poor medicine and shows lack of compassion.

Conventional Prescribing

The very term painkillers sounds appealing and comforting. Most doctors readily reach for their prescription pad when the patient mentions any degree of discomfort. There are probably hundreds of prescription-only medications that are said to tackle pain, though only a couple of dozen are regularly chosen.

That's as far as most doctors will go; few look for any real causes and they have a battery of off-the-cuff diagnoses that mean they will not have to do a work-up on the case: things like lumbago, myalgia (which means nothing), fibrositis (which means even less), dysmenorrhea, arthritis, a touch of sciatica and—if all else fails—it's your age, Mrs. Jones.

But there are plenty of over-the-counter options, you will say. It's hardly worth going to the doctor, except for tougher degrees of pain. There are hundreds of those to choose from, too.

It will surprise you when I say there are really only two pain-control drugs you ever need to consider: aspirin or morphine. If a significant dose of aspirin does not stop the pain, your doctor should switch to morphine. It's as simple as that.

Note that both are from natural plant sources and each has a long and honorable history. Anything to the contrary is just disinformation, bad science and poor clinical skills.

Less Choice Than You Think

The truth is that almost all pain drugs (let's use the term analgesics, meaning "takes away pain") are just derivatives of these two classes of substances, derived from plant families. Aspirin or opiates. I introduce panadol/tylenol here as the "other aspirin".

You know how drug corporations like to make money by tweaking a simple molecule, patenting their new "invention" and then selling it for a fortune. Since aspirin (salicylic acid) and morphine are basic plant molecules, they cannot be patented and paracetamol/acetaminophen is long out of patent, so pharmaceutical companies don't take them seriously.

Instead they waste their ingenuity coming up with variants that can be patented and sold at enormous profit.

Aspirin (salicylic acid)

This, along with penicillin, must be one of the most famous medicinal substances of all time! It began life centuries ago as a folk herbal con-coction, taken from the bark of the willow tree *Salyx alba* (white wil-low). Only in the nineteenth century did "aspirin" tablets become avail-able. The Egyptians and Hippocrates knew this remedy well, especially as a way to reduce fevers.

Aspirin's popularity declined after the development of acetamino-phen/paracetamol (Tylenol, Panadol) in 1956 and ibuprofen in 1962. Now there are legion alternative painkillers on the market, enough to easily confuse a patient in need of help. But as the inherent toxicity of these "safe" alternatives has become known, aspirin is making some-thing of a comeback.

The big story is that aspirin is supposed to cause gastric irritation and intestinal bleeding. It does; but I'm sure this propensity is grossly exag-gerated by aggressive marketing from competitor substances (which in turn emerge as not at all safe).

The problem is the classic one: salicylic acid is so old-fashioned there can be no patent for it. That means drug companies cannot make their fat profits. So they denigrate it, bring out their own patented molecules that last for a time and then, when found toxic, they are withdrawn.

To try and juice up profits a little with the simple stuff, pharmaceutical manufacturers have taken to "designer" aspirin and derivatives, such as mixtures of paracetamol and caffeine or aspirin and paracetamol com-bined. There are then pushed with fancy advertising campaigns.

The truth is, you can forget all these nonsense brands and go for one product: soluble aspirin. The easily-dissolved version causes far less gastric irritation and is probably the safest of all the over-the-counter painkillers.

If you are sensitive to salicylates, then use ordinary paracetamol/acetaminophen (Panadol/Tylenol). Just don't kid yourself it's "safe" (section 3). Make sure your doctor monitors liver health carefully.

The Opioids Group

The name of this class of drugs derives from the opium poppy (*Papaver somniferum*). The three principle active compounds in the poppy extract are morphine, papaverine, and codeine. Heroin is a synthetic derivative.

You will probably also know the term *narcotic*: "narcosis" simply means being put to sleep, but the word narcotic has nasty overtones in modern society.

The first opiates are believed to have been cultivated during the Neolithic period in what is now known as Switzerland. The Sumerians used opium, nearly 6000 years ago. Hippocrates, the father of modern medicine, prescribed opium (2,500 years ago) and so did the great Roman physician Galen (2,000 years ago).

In other words, these are not new compounds.

By the nineteenth century, opium had become probably the most popular drug in the world and was widely used throughout Europe in a number of forms, such as laudanum and opium. Historically the British fought the Chinese for the right to continue exporting opium to China, via Hong Kong, and at that time opium was officially and quite legally imported into Britain.

All the active opiate derivatives work in a similar way, which is that they produce pain relief by creating a sense of detachment rather than actually blocking pain sensations.

Only recently has it been realized that opiates such as morphine and heroin work simply and solely because they imitate 20 so natural painkiller substances found in our bodies, the endorphins and the enkephalins, so-called.

Our endorphins give us that familiar warm, comfortable fuzzy feeling. Indeed, the reason an addict feels so desperate and ill is that continued use of the drugs tricks the brain into discontinuing production of natural endorphins. Without these feel-good compounds life is very miserable. Cold turkey is very hard.

Endorphins, the natural on-board painkillers, are produced by our body whenever it needs to overcome pain in order to survive. So, for example, a caveman being chased by a sabre-tooth tiger and at risk of his life might slip and sprain an ankle, yet will hardly feel the injury and will go on running until he escapes. Only then will the pain become noticeable.

This works in a positive environment too, such as a sports game where there has been a degree of bruising and injury. The body will produce its own endorphins in order that the player can largely ignore the discomfort and continue with a high level of involvement in the match. Again only when the game is over will the endorphin production cease and then the player becomes aware of pain.

Disambiguation:

Laudanum is the name for an old-fashioned morphine preparation that is no longer available (there are recipes for it on the Internet but beware: it's illegal).

Heroin is also known as diamorphine (two molecules of morphine stuck together). It is thus more potent than morphine. It was originally thought to be non-addictive but that is very obviously not true.

Codeine is a milder analgesic, for tougher headaches perhaps, but is definitely in the opium group. Like all opiates, it causes intestinal slowing.

Methadone is a completely synthetic opioid (meaning like an opiate but not an opiate). It was originally produced by the German pharmaceutical company Axis during the second world war and marketed as "Dolophine" (to honor Adolph Hitler). Today it's rarely used as a painkiller but mainly as an aid to curing opiate addiction.

Kaolin and morphine mixture (*mist. kaolin et morph*). You have heard of this and may be wondering about the morphine part. This medicine contains a low dose of morphine—not enough to have any analgesic benefit—and is used purely for its anti-diarrheal effect. It works directly on opiate receptors that are found in the muscles lining the intestinal walls.

You couldn't drink enough of the stuff to get a high, so forget it! You'll clog your guts, that's all.

Other Opiates

Opioid medications may be administered orally, by injection, via nasal mucosa or oral mucosa, rectally (suppository), transdermally, intravenously, epidurally, or intrathecally.

Morphine is the gold standard to which all narcotics are compared.

Fentanyl has the benefit of less histamine release and thus fewer side effects. It can also be administered via transdermal patch, which is convenient for chronic pain management.

Oxycodone is used across the Americas and Europe for relief of serious chronic pain; its main slow-release formula is known as OxyContin, and short-acting tablets, capsules, syrups and ampoules are available, making it suitable for acute intractable pain or breakthrough pain.

Pethidine, known in North America as meperidine, is not the best for pain management due to its low potency, short duration of action, and toxicity associated with repeated use. It has a long tradition in midwifery, as it is considered to be less dangerous to the fetus, once born.

Pentazocine, dextromoramide, and dipipanone are also not recommended in new patients except for acute pain where other analgesics are not tolerated or are inappropriate, for pharmacological and misuse-related reasons.

In chronic pain conditions, a combination of a long-acting or extended release opioid is often prescribed in conjunction with a shorter-acting opioid (oxycodone, morphine, or hydromorphone) for breakthrough pain or exacerbations.

Methadone is paradoxical in that it can be used as an effective analgesic but is also used for the treatment of opioid addiction/detoxification, which it does by blocking morphine receptors.

Other than this outline, patients or their family really don't need more technical data.

The Problem of Addiction

Doctors are reluctant to prescribe opioids in adequate amounts, in the mistaken belief they will lead inevitably to addiction. Because the patient is given inadequate doses, he or she may believe the injections are "not working". Moreover, doctors will often not prescribe the drugs for as long a period as needed. This is bad medicine and totally misguided.

Incidentally, heroin and morphine are virtually identical in effect and Dr. Robert Twycross, who has worked at St Christopher's Hospice in London and the Churchill Hospital Oxford, has shown conclusively that neither patients nor doctors can observe any difference between the two substances. This is also backed up by an American study carried out at the Memorial Sloan-Kettering Cancer Center in New York, where Dr. Stanley Wallenstein showed over a series of 24 cancer patients with post-operative pain, and another 46 with chronic pain, that heroin was neither better nor worse than morphine.

Both are very good indeed; no question. So why are they not used enough?

In 1961, the world community adopted an international agreement—the 1961 Single Convention on Narcotic Drugs—that proclaimed "narcotic drugs…indispensible for the relief of pain and suffering" and instructed countries to make adequate provision to ensure their availability for medical needs. Today, almost fifty years later, the promise of that agreement remains largely unfulfilled, particularly—but not only—in low- and middle-income countries. In September 2008, the World Health Organization (WHO) estimated that approximately 80 percent of the world population has either no or insufficient access to treatment for moderate to severe pain and that every year tens of millions of people around the world, including around 4 million cancer patients and 0.8 million HIV/AIDS patients at the end of their lives suffer from such pain without treatment. ["Please, do not make us suffer any more..." Access to pain treatment as a human right. New York: Human Rights Watch; March 2009:1.]

The concern is always that patients will become addicted, if they are given medical morphine or heroin in significant doses. After all, it's a deadly street drug and gets people really hooked; don't we all know that? Under-treatment may be due to physicians' fear of being accused of over-prescribing.

Under-Treatment

However, as a result of two recent cases in California, where physicians who failed to provide adequate pain relief were successfully sued for "elder abuse," the North American medical and health care communities appear to be undergoing a shift in perspective.

According to Human Rights Watch, pain relief is a right; moreover, pain treatment has to be free from cruel, inhuman, and degrading treatment. That includes being spared from under-treatment.

Under-treatment, in the elderly in particular, can be due to a variety of reasons, including the misconception that pain is a normal part of aging, therefore it is unrealistic to expect older adults to be pain-free. It is often supposed that older adults have decreased pain sensitivity, especially if they have a cognitive dysfunction such as dementia and that opioids should not be administered to older adults, as they are too dangerous. However, with appropriate assessment and careful administration and monitoring, older adults can have the same level of pain management as any other population of care.

The federal Center for Medicare and Medicaid Services has declared a willingness to charge health care providers with fraud if they accept payment for providing adequate pain relief while failing to do so. Thus clinical practice guidelines and standards are evolving into clear, unambiguous statements on acceptable pain management, so health care providers, in California at least, can no longer avoid culpability by claiming that poor or no pain relief meets community standards. [Weissman V, Martin MD. The legal liability of under-treatment of pain. *Education Resource Center.* Jan–Feb 2001; 6(3): 15–24.]

The addiction from medical usage of opiates is, in fact, a complete myth. If you are in a lot of pain, don't hesitate. It turns out that a person in pain will not become addicted when treated with these rather superior drugs or only extremely rarely. Available evidence shows this quite conclusively. For example, in the Yom-Kippur War (1973) it was found that, although thousands of injured Israeli soldiers had been given morphine, only one had become addicted. Those are good odds, if you are in dreadful pain.

Such observations fit well with conclusion that it is the personality of the patient and the circumstances in which he or she is found will dictate becoming an addict, not the substance itself. In other words *there is nothing inherently present in morphine or heroin that is bound to result in addiction*. That's probably why they were first used in the belief they were not addictive.

Demand it in sufficient dosage, if you need it (if aspirin at full dose won't hold the pain). But of course demand also a solution to the cause of the problem!

Tranquillizers

Now let's look at another class of drugs that is often called upon to help with pain: tranquillizers, especially the benzodiazepines (Valium family). These are not analgesics at all. The idea (a rather silly one) is the hope that by relaxing the patient, he or she will cope with pain better.

The trouble is that commonly used tranquillizers—a misnomer anyway—are highly addictive in their own right. And they do have fierce long-term side effects, most notably tardive dyskinesia. More of that in a moment.

First introduced in the early 1960s, the benzodiazepines include several well-known brand names, such as Valium and Ativan. Over the next two or three decades, these drugs rose to become the most widely used prescription drugs in the world and, by wildly overprescribing them, doctors have produced the world's biggest drug addiction problem.

These compounds were originally supposed to be short-term aids for suffering and anxiety, but many doctors began to use them as multipurpose drugs and hand them out to patients when they could think of nothing else to give.

Their use in pain control is based on the fact that patients suffering pain are often anxious and depressed and frequently have difficulty getting to sleep at night. However, since the pain is the cause of the anxiety and depression, not the other way round, this explanation for their value does not hold water.

Secondly, doctors prescribe tranquillizers for a self-serving reason, which is that, when they themselves are frustrated and don't know how to deal with the case, they find that the tranquillizers will make the patients sleepy, more cooperative, and less complaining. The problem is that these are amongst the most addictive drugs of all. The United States Senate health committee testifying in Washington in 1979 said that tranquillizers were America's number one drug problem apart from alcohol. This is saying they are far worse and more addictive then so-called "heavy drugs."

It is said to be harder to get off the tranquilizer habit then it is to kick heroin or morphine. Ironically patients in severe pain would be better being prescribed morphine which is less addictive than tranquillizers, the latter having no effect on the pain and so solving nothing.

In fact, one experiment conducted at the behavior research laboratory in Washington University found that diazepam (Valium) was shown to make some patients more sensitive to pain. This, of course, is absurdly counter-productive.

The long-term horror that emerged from excessive use of benzodiazepine drugs is a difficult-to-treat and often incurable form of muscle dysfunction called tardive dyskinesia ("tardive" just means delayed onset). It is characterized by involuntary, repetitive body movements.

It may improve by simply stopping the medication, but this rarely happens. Indeed, the patient may have been off the drug for many years before the onset of the characteristic neurological deterioration.

Some examples of these types of involuntary movements include grimaces, tongue movements, lip smacking and puckering; excessive eye blinking and rapid, involuntary movements of the limbs, torso, and fingers may also occur.

Some individuals become so incapacitated that they cannot walk effectively. But neither can the person remain still. This is the opposite of Parkinson's disease; Parkinson's patients have difficulty getting moving, whereas tardive dyskinesia patients have difficulty not moving.

Drugs similar to dopamine, the classic treatment for Parkinsonism, have been tried, with little to celebrate. Basically, it's an incurable degenerative tragedy.

Drugs other than benzodiazepines which may cause tardive dyskinesia are, for example: chlorpromazine (Thorazine), haloperidol (Haldol), olanzapine (Zyprexa), prochlorperazine (Compazine), paliperidone (Invega), and risperidone (Risperdal).

The price to pay, in my opinion, is too high to make the use of any tranquillizer or anti-psychotic medication justifiable.

The imperative instead is to find and adopt natural, holistic, and more healing approaches to pain and other mental difficulties.

Anti-Depressants

Drugs of this class were originally developed to treat depression (obviously). But some physicians feel they have a place in pain management. For example, Amitriptyline is often prescribed for chronic muscular pain in the arms, legs, neck, and lower back.

I am less certain of the value of anti-depressants. Nor do I like the attitude that being in constant pain is by nature very depressing. That does not make it primary. Moreover, anti-depressants have their own (often severe and incapacitating) side effects. These may become permanent.

It would be far better to properly resolve the pain condition than smother it with layers of soporific and mood-altering drugs. I think the use of anti-depressants has a pejorative overtone, somewhat implying the patient is at fault whereas, in my view, the attendant physician is the one at fault, being ineffective.

It could also encourage laziness in the attendant practitioner, meaning he or she may take the view that the misery is now "solved" and they don't have to continue looking for an effective approach.

There is one justification: antidepressants may promote sleep, which can be difficult when you are in pain.

Steroids

Since the 1950s, this class of drugs has been a huge temptation for doctors to prescribe. They certainly work and sometimes work very well. But the spin-off and side effects can be very considerable and make the gamble somewhat risky.

Let me clarify: by steroids, I mean corticosteroid substances. These are so named because they are hormones secreted by the adrenal cortex, the outer layer of those glands (adrenalin or epinephrine comes from the adrenal core or medulla).

I'm not talking about anabolic (body-building) steroids, which are bad for a different reason. The main effect of corticosteroids is to block inflammation. They do this, in turn, by blocking the proper working of the immune system. The average reader will easily see the apparent benefit of stopping inflammation. But it is only an apparent advantage because we need inflammation, wherever it occurs.

The problem is not the inflammatory process; that's the body's own defense. Inflammation is necessary and protective. The problem is with the agents that cause inflammation: the microbes, the toxic metals, the allergies, the chemical pollutants, and so on.

In fact, it's a very bad idea to hold inflammation in check and that's one of the big worries when prescribing steroidal compounds. We need our immune system to defend us from infections, for example. Without a proper response, we could not successfully fight off TB, salmonella, mumps, measles, and so on.

There are a number of other disadvantages with steroids. They thin our bones, cause the skin to stretch and become less supportive of tissues underneath, there is a strange distribution of weight gain, with lots of fat around the body but thin arms and legs, like sticks. They also mess up sugar metabolism and there can be serious mood swings.

None of this is good news. But there are times, as I said, when doctors may want to take the risk. If a person is suffering severe or intractable pain, relief at any cost may be preferable to continued suffering.

But once started, we encounter yet another problem with this class of drugs: they can't easily be stopped. To just discontinue taking corticosteroids will likely result in an unpleasant effect called a "rebound," where the symptoms come back worse than ever.

This leads to doctors trying to balance between too much drug and too many side effects or not taking enough, so that the benefit is not very pronounced. Again, as with doctors trying to hold back morphine-type drugs, the patient on steroids is between a rock and a hard place: he or she gets the worst of both aspects, rather than the best of both.

Certainly, if there is to be an attempt to cut down or cease taking corticosteroids, you need professional help and guidance. Steroid management skills are not common among primary care doctors and the matter may have to go to a rheumatologist or other specialist.

The commonest corticosteroid prescribed is prednisolone. It is a synthetic pharmaceutical and very powerful. That means first in side effects too. The typical dose is around 5 mg. But, for a severe eruption of pain and inflammation, large doses of up to 25 – 35 mg, or even higher, may be tried in desperation.

The trouble is, that difficulty of getting the dose back down again, without a severe rebound effect.

Topical applications may help; for example, creams and ointments can confine the therapeutic action to the skin; inhalers can speed prednisolone to the lungs, while sparing the rest of the body.

Corticosteroids can also be used to inject "hot spots," such as tendinitis or an inflamed joint. The drug is injected directly into the joint space. Occasionally they are offered as an epidural injection; that means outside the linings of the spinal cord but close enough to quench inflammation, at least temporarily.

Other injection techniques, such as biopuncture (section 9) and neural therapy are much to be preferred, since they are not weighed down by the same dangers and tend to harness Nature's own recovery systems.

If you are faced with long-term use of corticosteroids, you need to talk to your doctor about ways to minimize side effects. Exercise can help reduce muscle weakness and osteoporosis risks. And taking calcium and vitamin D supplements and prescription bone-building drugs can minimize bone thinning due to corticosteroids. You may need to reduce the number of calories you eat or increase your physical activity to prevent weight gain.

But there is no question: changing your diet and getting rid of inflammatory foods plus detoxing inflammatory metals and xenobiotic chemicals in your body can produce considerable improvement and may obviate any need for this heavy-handed class of drugs.

See section: 32

NSAIDs (Non-Steroidal Anti-Inflammatory Drugs)

This is the final class of drug likely to be commonly encountered in the control of pain. They are not analgesics but, as their name implies, they have an anti-inflammatory effect, even though they are not steroidal in nature.

NSAIDs comprise a large class of drugs with many different options. In addition to aspirin, there are currently several types of both non-prescription (over-the-counter) NSAIDs and prescription brands of NSAIDs. The three types of NSAIDs most commonly used to treat musculo-skeletal pain include:

- Ibuprofen (e.g., brand names Advil, Motrin, Nuprin)
- Naproxen (e.g., brand names Aleve, Naprosyn)
- COX-2 inhibitors (e.g., brand name Celebrex)

They do work (somewhat). The question is: are they safe to do what we want them to do? Vioxx, a notorious member of this class of drugs, killed at least 60,000 people before Merck removed it from the market; other estimates put the total far higher, at around 150,000. At least one independent source has estimated that 500,000 might be a more accurate figure, when taking into account the fact that a large number of elderly patients that died might have been certified as having a natural heart attack and no connection made with the fact they were taking Vioxx.

Certainly, the US death rate dropped by 100,000 per year, once Vioxx was taken off the market. That's a deadly result for merely treating pain.

Ibuprofen-Type (e.g., Advil, Motrin, Nuprin)

Ibuprofen was one of the original non-steroidal anti-inflammatory drugs and is available without a prescription.

For patients with musculo-skeletal pains, including mild or moderate back pain, tenderness, inflammation, and stiffness, or cervical spondylitis, ibuprofen is the most commonly recommended drug.

It does have some aspirin-like effects on the stomach, so people with active ulcers or sensitive stomachs should avoid ibuprofen. It is best to take ibuprofen with food to minimize the chance of stomach upset.

Ibuprofen also has a mild blood thinning effect that lasts a few hours, and can reduce the effectiveness of some blood pressure medications and diuretics (water pills), so care is needed.

The typical recommended dose for ibuprofen is 400mg taken every eight hours. Prescription doses can be as high as 800mg of ibuprofen every eight hours.

Naproxen-Type (e.g. Aleve, Naprosyn, Anaprox, Naprelan)

Naproxen is available in both non-prescription strength (e.g., brand name Aleve) and prescription strength (e.g., brand name Naprosyn).

For patients with musculo-skeletal pain, it works by reducing proteins that cause inflammation.

Naproxen also thins the blood, so individuals taking oral blood thinners or anticoagulants should avoid naproxen, as excessive blood thinning may lead to bleeding.

Naproxen also can have some adverse gastrointestinal side effects, so people with active ulcers or sensitive stomachs should avoid it. It is best to take naproxen with food to reduce the chance of upset stomach.

The usual adult dose is 250 to 500 mg twice daily using regular naproxen tablets.

COX-2 Inhibitors (e.g., Prescription Brand Celebrex)

This is a newer class of NSAID, which included the infamous Vioxx. The popular current brand name is Celebrex.

They are said to cause less gastro-intestinal disturbance and cause less blood clotting complications and are therefore safer for patients taking warfarin (Coumadin).

However, as Vioxx revealed, they have a disposition to potentially increase the risk for cardiovascular events, such as heart attack and stroke. The FDA has called for further research.

COX stands for, a group of enzymes (COX-1 and COX-2) that are responsible for the formation of a number of inflammatory substances, including prostaglandins (section 2). COX inhibition will therefore reduce the number of inflammatory substances circulating in the body. COX-2 does not seem to harm gastric mucosa.

So far so good, but drugs that selectively inhibit COX-2 do not seem to negate potentially dangerous side effects of NSAIDs, most notably an increased risk of renal failure, heart attack, thrombosis, and stroke. Vioxx, as I said, was eventually withdrawn, but other COX-2 selective NSAIDs, such as celecoxib, and etoricoxib, are still on the market.

Natural COX Inhibition

There are a number of cheap and effective natural COX inhibitors that surely make more sense than using a potentially lethal class of drugs.

Most notable are the omega-3 essential fatty acids (EFAs), from flax-seed, fish oils, or krill. Specific beneficial EFAs are eicosapentanoic acid (EPA) and docosahexaenoic acid (DHA), the latter more than the former. Fish do not naturally produce EPA, but obtain it from the algae they consume. EPA is converted to DHA in the body. DHA is a primary structural component of the human brain, cerebral cortex, skin, sperm, testicles, and retina.

Fish oils (e.g., cod liver oil) have been proposed as a reasonable alternative for the treatment of rheumatoid arthritis and other conditions as a consequence of the fact that they provide less cardiovascular risk than other treatments including NSAIDs.

Culinary mushrooms, like maitake, may be able to partially inhibit COX-2 enzymes.

A variety of flavonoids, the highly colored plant antioxidants we have all become used to, have been found to inhibit COX-2.

Hyperforin, from St. John's wort, has been shown to inhibit COX-1 around 3-18 times as much as aspirin. A better choice.

Resveratrol. I found several studies showing that this important compound helps reduce COX function. You can take it as a supplement (it's not stable) or drink the wine! Up to you.

Calcitriol (vitamin D) significantly inhibits the expression of the COX-2 gene.

Curcumin is the active ingredient in turmeric, the yellow powder found in curry. Curcumin is being extensively investigated for its anticancer and anti-inflammatory properties. It also helps to improve circulation and prevent blood clotting. Turmeric has been used in traditional medicines for easing the pain of sprains, strains, bruises, and joint inflammation, as well as for treating skin and digestive issues.

If you are not already in the habit of enjoying good curries, get to know them. I've been saying for nearly 40 years that Indian curries are mainly good whole food: nothing in the cook pot but vegetables, meats, and spices! Just stay away from the naan bread and chapatis and you won't get fat!

Most curcumin supplements that are commercially available contain far less than the proper therapeutic serving necessary to deliver powerful health benefits. Inferior curcumin supplements have flooded the market—and many of them contain only 4% actives, and the rest consists of maltodextrin or other food additives.

Make sure the product you buy is free of padding ingredients and contains at least 700 mg. Most commercially available curcumin supplements contain only 450 mg to 500 mg.

Choose only full-spectrum curcumin. That means it contains not only curcumin extract (with 95% curcuminoids) but it also contains pure whole turmeric root full-spectrum powder—which means it can be readily absorbed by the body.

Both curcumin extract and turmeric root must be organic. Typical commercially-grown is nutritionally depleted and filled with pesticides. Make sure the curcumin supplement is manufactured by a certified supplier. In the USA, look for a label that says according to "current good manufacturing practices" (cGMP). This means all raw ingredients and finished products are tested for purity, safety, strength and quality.

Otherwise you are on your own; note the majority of supplement manufacturers are not cGMP-compliant!

Other Drugs That Impact Pain

Sometimes other substances have an incidental (indirect) effect on pain or may help analgesics combat various types of pain and parts of the overall pain experience, and are hence called adjuvant medications. *Adjuvant* means: an ingredient (as in a prescription or a solution) that modifies the action of the principal ingredient; something (as a drug or method) that enhances the effectiveness of medical treatment.

For example, Gabapentin—an anti-epileptic—not only exerts effects alone on neuropathic pain, but it can also potentiate opiates. [Zogopoulos P, Vasileiou I, Patsouris E, Theocharis SE. The role of endocannabinoids in pain modulation. *Fundam Clin Pharmacol.* Feb 2013; 27(1): 64–80.]

While perhaps not prescribed as such, other drugs such as Tagamet (cimetidine) and even simple grapefruit juice may also potentiate opiates by inhibiting the cytochrome P450 enzymes in the liver, thereby slowing metabolism of the drug.

Tagamet has its own specific pain relief mode in certain types of migraine.

In addition, orphenadrine, cyclobenzaprine, trazodone, and other drugs with anticholinergic properties are useful in conjunction with opioids for neuropathic pain. Orphenadrine and cyclobenzaprine are also muscle relaxants, and therefore particularly useful in painful musculoskeletal conditions.

Clonidine has found use as an analgesic for this same purpose, and all of the mentioned drugs potentiate the effects of opioids overall.

PARACETAMOL

Paracetamol (acetaminophen) is sometimes thought of as the "other aspirin." The perception is that it's a safer alternative; it doesn't result in gastric bleeding, like its salicylate brother.

Panadol (UK) or Tylenol (USA) is often the first resort for any pain, from a toothache to arthritis. But it's not so safe, after all.

Here's an example of the difference between UK informed public attitudes and the American mass ignorance that doesn't seem to care, until Big Brother tells it what to think.

People in the UK have long been aware that a paracetamol overdose can kill. That goes back to 1998, when the government restricted the number of tablets that could be bought in one purchase and ran an information campaign explaining the change. The measures prevent an estimated 1000 deaths a year.

US awareness is much lower. When investigative journalism group Propublica revealed in 2013 that 1500 Americans die annually from accidental overdoses of Tylenol, it was apparently big news!

Paracetamol poisoning is responsible for nearly 80,000 visits to the emergency room in the US each year, and a third of these are people who overdosed accidentally.

Although pill packets clearly state that the maximum recommended dose is no more than 3 or 4 grams spread over 24 hours (or six to eight 500 mg tablets), some people take more than this, thinking it's safe.

Is It Worth the Risk?

Its technical name is N-acetyl-p-aminophenol and paracetamol/acetaminophen is on the first rung of the World Health Organization's "analgesic ladder" for cancer pain control. We spoon it to our children to fight fever, as adults we swallow it to relieve headaches or period cramps, and as we get older we're prescribed it to soothe arthritis or backache.

In the US, 27 billion doses of paracetamol/acetaminophen are sold each year, and it is found in more than 600 products.

Paracetamol was discovered in the late 19th century, but didn't become an immediate hit. It really took off in the 1960s, in response to emerging concerns about the long-term side effects of aspirin and other non-steroidal anti-inflammatory drugs (NSAIDs). Today in the US, there are about 16,500 NSAID-related deaths a year in people with arthritis alone.

We think of it as a safe alternative to aspirin. Sure, if taken in larger doses, it can damage your liver or kidneys. But otherwise, at the recommended dose, it's fine, right?

Maybe not. It's emerging that long-term use has significant hazards that may displace it is as the number one "safe" starter analgesic. Taken over a period, it can damage the stomach as much as NSAIDs. That might be an acceptable risk in exchange for pain relief.

But— paracetamol/acetaminophen doesn't really work all that well, apparently. More on that shortly.

Long-Term Dosing

In 2011, Michael Doherty of Nottingham City Hospital, UK, published a study that was hard to ignore. He followed the progress of 892 men and women with the niggling knee pain that often sets in at middle age, often an early symptom of osteoarthritis. Some patients were given paracetamol, others ibuprofen, while a third and fourth group were given either a high- or low-dose combination of the two.

When Doherty looked at the blood results of those taking it, he was surprised to find that levels of hemoglobin were dropping fast. What's more, patients' red blood cells were growing smaller and paler. Taken together, these signs are a sure indication that hidden bleeding is taking place.

In fact, after just three months, a fifth of the patients had lost the equivalent of an entire unit of blood (about 15 ounces or 450 milliliters). That was the same degree of loss as found in those taking ibuprofen – only the ibuprofen group reported feeling less pain. [*Annals of the Rheumatic Diseases*. 70: 1534.]

Even more startling, when combining high doses of both paracetamol and ibuprofen, the hemoglobin loss after three months jumped to *two units* of blood. That suggests to me that the main site of bleeding is different for each drug.

It's still bad news for paracetamol's safety record.

The upshot: When taken for long periods, paracetamol/acetaminophen may be just as damaging to the stomach lining as NSAID drugs are.

Liver Toxicity

Even worse, if you regularly exceed 4 g (8 tablets) a day, you can quickly encounter serious liver complications, even in healthy people. Moreover, if the liver is already compromised, due to alcoholism or non-alcoholic fatty liver disease (NAFLD), even less of the drug can be dangerous.

Let me point out, if you don't already know, that over 40% of the US population over the age of 65 has NAFLD. For them, even the "recommended" safe dose it too high.

Even so, it's still with us. The UK's National Institute for Health and Care Excellence (NICE), the body that sets standards for medical practice, still recommends paracetamol/acetaminophen as the first-choice drug for treating the chronic pain associated with conditions like osteoarthritis and lower back pain. The American College of Rheumatology also recommends it for arthritis.

If paracetamol/acetaminophen really was effective against chronic pain, you might consider the trade-off worthwhile, but the drug has been found seriously wanting. A review of research that looked at people taking paracetamol/acetaminophen to relieve chronic joint pain found seven studies that compared the drug with a placebo. Five of these found it to be marginally more effective, but two found no difference.

In other words, here we have a drug that's toxic and doesn't even do what it's supposed to do. Contrast that with aspirin, which is risky but definitely worthwhile for pain relief.

In March, the Osteoarthritis Research Society International changed its paracetamol guidelines to "uncertain" to reflect growing safety concerns. And, for a while at least, it looked like these concerns would be similarly heeded in the UK.

When NICE issued new draft guidelines for osteoarthritis in August 2013, it did away with the recommendation of paracetamol as a first resort and flagged its potential dangers. "On balance, the risks of paracetamol outweigh the benefits of any gain in symptom control," the report read.

Yet, by the time the final version was published in February 2014, the old advice had been reinstated. This was partly down to objections raised by doctors about having few alternative options, though NICE says it is also awaiting the results of a more comprehensive review of over-the-counter painkillers by the UK's Medicines and Healthcare Products Regulatory Agency.

A triumph of baloney over reason.

Number Needed to Treat

Pharmacists measure the effectiveness of painkillers by looking at whether they can reduce the reported sensation of pain by at least 50 per cent and by counting how many people would need to take it for one person to experience this level of relief compared with placebo. This is known as the number needed to treat (NNT).

For example, in the case of the moderate pain of a sprained ankle, 3.8 people would need to take a standard 1 g dose of paracetamol (2 tablets) for one of them to get effective relief. For a standard 400-milligram dose of ibuprofen, the NNT is 2.5. That means that paracetamol is 35% less effective as a painkiller.

Bottom line: With paracetamol, if it's not going to work within a week, it's never going to work for you. Tylenol's US drug label clearly states that consumers should stop use and ask a doctor if they have pain that gets worse or lasts more than 10 days.

Should you toss it from your medicine cabinet? No. I think for short-lived aches and pains, if you follow the instructions and if you don't take it in too-large doses, paracetamol is relatively safe.

But for ongoing pain, it may be time to start looking for alternatives. That's what this book is about.

ANTIBIOTICS COULD BE SURPRISE PAINKILLERS!

Bacteria flood our bodies and may be the real cause of arthritis.

You may or may not know that joint inflammation these days is often seen as directly due to micro-organisms within the joint itself. Bacteria get in there, raise hell, resulting in inflammation and pain, and we call it "arthritis." It has little to do with age and "wear-and-tear," which is the medical school model!

This realization that an actual physical infection leads to arthritis is relatively new. Over the years, I've cured thousands of arthritis cases, using the food allergy/elimination approach. So, how could that be? It's not counter-intuitive. If you eliminate stress foods, the immune system recovers from the overload and is better able to deal with the invader germs. Less joint inflammation is the result.

Remember my lifetime saying, that you don't need zero burden to get zero symptoms; you just have to reduce the overload to the point where the body can cope. Step back within the threshold limits and the body recovers.

Anyway, a new controversy has erupted from this topic. Dr. Hanne B. Albert and colleagues of the Spine Centre of Southern Denmark have found that a significant number of back pain sufferers will benefit from a course of antibiotics.

Of course, Dr. Albert's colleagues are stupefied and attack her relentlessly because her finding "cannot be true." Nobody these days seems interested in what actually works, just what fits in with current dogma. The dogma is more important than clinical results, per se.

Not that dogma has much to offer back pain sufferers. Recommended orthodox treatments include painkillers, hot or cold compresses, physical therapy, keeping active, and (rarely) lifestyle changes.

In extreme cases, when other treatments have failed, surgery may be recommended and the patient is told this is the only option left. In my working life, I have never met a single patient who benefitted from back surgery—but I have met a good many who have been permanently ruined by these procedures!

Danish Study Rocks

In the first study of 61 patients who had spinal surgery for lower back pain, the researchers found bacteria in 46% of the slipped discs.

The work of Albert et al. validates and builds on previous work by Alistair Stirling and colleagues (and others), who found Propionibacterium acnes, a normal skin organism, in degenerated lumbar intervertebral discs.

The research team recruited 162 patients who had been living with low back pain for more than six months following a slipped disc. Half of the patients were given a 100-day course of antibiotic treatment, while the others received a placebo.

The back-pain sufferers were randomized into two groups: a placebo group, and a group given antibiotics daily for 100 days. Result: Patients who took the antibiotics improved on all outcome measures, in statistically highly significant fashion, not only at the end of 100 days but one year later.

The findings were published in the *European Spine Journal*.

Resistance to a Cure

As I said, the run-of-the-mill underperforming doctors are incensed by this suggestion. Media reports that antibiotics could be a cure for back pain have alarmed John O'Dowd, a consultant spinal surgeon and president of the British Society for Back Pain Research.

"Unless you've had a disc herniation ... I don't think you should be getting too excited, and I don't think this is going to be a treatment for you," O'Dowd says. "I think this is another useful building block of evidence, but I don't think it's either a cure or the answer to back pain."

Well, the spinal surgery that he does is certainly a disaster. But it pays the mortgage, even if it doesn't help patients.

Where Do the Bacteria Come from?

The answer may surprise you. They come from anaerobic mouth and skin commensal organisms during normal bacteremias (bacteria in the blood).

Oh yes, didn't I mention? Bacteria are swimming around in our blood all the time! Subclinical episodes of bacteremia are not uncommon; in fact they are normal. The typical entry point for bacteria arriving in the blood is the periodontal space (and/or the gums themselves, in the case of gingivitis). You don't have to have periodontal disease or gingivitis to experience bacteremia, however. Any dental procedure, even vigorous brushing of the teeth, poses the risk of a bacteremic event.

Bacteremia is also possible when boils (pimples, carbuncles) are traumatized, whether deliberately (through incision) or accidentally (e.g., by shaving). Obviously, any open skin wound is also an invitation to bacteremia.

Bacteremia is also a common complication in urinary tract infections.

These "normal bacteremias" are short-lived.

But even a "normal" bacteremia can lead to trouble, because once bacteria enter the blood, they look for areas of inflammation in which to congregate and take up residence. So for example: catheters, implants, sore joints, slipped discs, and inflamed coronary arteries are all potential sites for bacterial occupancy. (Take note: the connection between periodontal disease and heart disease is well established. After adjusting for age, sex, diabetes status, serum total cholesterol, smoking, and hypertension, death rate for coronary heart disease goes up by a factor of two for people with gingivitis or missing teeth.)

What it means is that if your gums bleed when you brush (or if you have a problem with boils or acne), you could (arguably) be at risk for a variety of ailments, from heart disease to arthritis to chronic lower back pain.

Where Is All This Leading?

I want you to grasp what I have been teaching my subscribers for years:

- We are up against a continuous pool of bacteria; they flood our bodies.
- Once out of control, they are potentially very deadly.
- They cannot be stopped by antibiotics (because of increasing resistance).
- You need to learn about alternatives to dangerous antibiotics.

That's the crux of this information; you need to learn about antibiotic alternatives and you need to learn NOW. The Golden Age of Antibiotics is over. Antibiotics are starting to fail.

In any case, it would be wise to know what you can do instead of drugs. That's obvious.

But what intrigues me is the possibility of cleansing your "normal bacteremias," gum disease, and back pains by using holistic ALTERNATIVES to antibiotics.

You know what? There are countless workable substitutes, mostly safe and certainly safe to use if you follow instructions.

Some natural plant substances actually out-perform modern high-power antibiotics. But do you know what these plant and food substances are?

You should!

To learn about this and some day save a life in your family, get my powerhouse reader describing lots of safe, natural, holistic alternatives to bugaboo antibiotics.

In my usual way, I have loaded the text with scientific references; this is not some old housewives' tale of what works and what doesn't.

To be armed with such knowledge, you are ready to face the future safely, instead of ending up a "statistic" from random septicemia.

Read about this massive compilation of antibiotics alternatives I have called "How to Survive in a World without Antibiotics." Go here:

PAIN SPECIALISTS AND PAIN CLINICS

The treatment of pain was traditionally a "Cinderella medicine," meaning it's little regarded and often starved for personnel and funds. The ruling attitude seemed to be that "pain is everyone's business but pain is no one's responsibility." Dr. Vernon Coleman has written that, "In too many hospitals the term pain clinic has been used to add dignity and hope to an outpatients' department with a long waiting list where a single overloaded specialist offers patients a straight choice between drug therapy and surgery."

In 1982, Dr. J. W. Lloyd of the Pain Relief Unit at Abingdon Hospital in Oxfordshire reported in the *Journal of the Royal Society of Medicine* that in the United Kingdom no less than 95 percent of all pain clinics were run by anesthetists, often working single-handed.

However, since 1993 that has changed. The World Institute of Pain (WIP), a worldwide organization founded in 1993, offers a fellowship program utilizing a global forum for education, training, and networking to qualified physicians in the field of Pain Medicine. In 2001, the WIP and its FIPP Board of Exam introduced the Fellow of Interventional Pain Practice (FIPP), a physician certification program by the FIPP Board of Examination. According to WIP, the purpose of the fellowship is global advancement and standardization of interventional pain practice. Over 800 physicians from 50 different countries have been FIPP-certified. [Mission statement concept and goals. World Institute of Pain Web site. http://www.worldinstituteofpain.org/site/pages.php?pageid=24. Accessed April 7, 2014.]

Now we have a significant number of pain clinics, geared solely to the management of pain, particularly the severe intractable kind.

History of the Concept

The original impetus came during World War II. Dr. John Bonica, a Sicilian-American anesthesiologist and chief of anesthesiology at a large military hospital in Fort Lewis, Washington, was confronted with 7,700 beds, regularly filled with young injured soldiers suffering from serious war injuries and concomitant pain.

Bonica's search became the quest to find effective methods of pain management.

In 1947, John left the Army and became Chief of Anesthesia at Tacoma General Hospital. He devoted his career to the study of pain, establishing it as a multidisciplinary field. He believed in a team approach to the field of pain management, incorporating various specialties to treat acute and chronic pain. He created residency programs, chaired departments, wrote standard texts in the field, and had his work published in numerous languages. In 1966, Bonica became president of the American Society of Anesthesiology.

His classic text, *The Management of Pain, Second Edition*, was published in 1990. Pope John Paul II requested to have a copy for his own personal library. Bonica's *Principles and Practice of Obstetric and Analgesic Anesthesia*—written as a result of the fact that his wife almost died of complications during the birth of their first child—became an enduring legacy used worldwide.

Today, pain clinics have an armory of tools. The typical pain management team includes medical practitioners, clinical psychologists, physiotherapists, occupational therapists, physician assistants, nurse practitioners, and clinical nurse specialists. [Main CJ, Spanswick C. Pain management: an interdisciplinary approach. Churchill Livingstone; 2000. ISBN 0-443-05683-8.]

Such a team may also include other mental-health specialists and massage therapists. Effective long-term management of pain may require interdisciplinary cooperation with all of these specialists and their different skill sets.

When a painful injury or pathology is resistant to treatment and persists, when pain persists after the injury or pathology has healed, and when medical science cannot identify the cause of pain, the task of medicine is to relieve suffering. Treatment modalities directed towards chronic pain include pharmacological measures, such as analgesics, tranquillizers or antidepressants; interventional procedures, such as surgery and ablation of nerves, physical therapy, physical exercise, or application of ice and/or heat; and psychological measures, such as biofeedback, hypnosis, and cognitive behavioral therapy.

Cognitive Behavioral Therapy

Cognitive behavioral therapy (CBT) for pain is supposed to help patients to understand the relationship between one's physiology (e.g., pain and muscle tension), thoughts, emotions, and behaviors. A main goal in treatment is cognitive restructuring to encourage helpful thought patterns, targeting a behavioral activation of healthy activities, such as regular exercise and pacing.

Lifestyle changes are also taught, to improve sleep patterns and to develop better coping skills for pain and other stressors using various techniques (e.g., relaxation, diaphragmatic breathing, and even biofeedback).

Studies have demonstrated the usefulness of cognitive behavioral therapy in the management of chronic low back pain, producing significant decreases in physical and psychosocial disability. A study published in the January 2012 issue of the *Archives of Internal Medicine* found that CBT is significantly more effective than standard care in the treatment of people with body-wide pain, like fibromyalgia.

Evidence for the usefulness of CBT in the management of adult chronic pain is generally poorly understood, due partly to the proliferation of techniques of doubtful quality and to the poor quality of reporting in clinical trials. The crucial content of individual interventions has not been isolated and the important contextual elements, such as therapist training and development of treatment manuals, have not been determined. The widely varying nature of the resulting data makes useful systematic review and meta-analysis within the field very difficult. [Pain management. Wikipedia Web site. http://en.wikipedia.org/wiki/Pain_management.]

In 2009, a systematic review of randomized controlled trials (RCTs) of psychological therapies for the management of adult chronic pain (excluding headache) found that CBT had "weak" effects in improving pain and minimal effects on disability associated with chronic pain. However, CBT was effective in altering mood outcomes and there is some evidence that these changes are maintained at six months.

The results, from the same study authors, regarding children, found more cheerful news: Psychological treatments are effective in pain control for children with headache and with musculoskeletal and recurrent abdominal pain. These results appeared to be maintained. There is some evidence available to estimate effects on disability or mood. [Eccleston C, Palermo TM, Williams AC, Lewandowski A, Morley S. Psychological therapies for the management of chronic and recurrent pain in children and adolescents. Cochrane Database Syst Rev (2). 2009; CD003968. doi:10.1002/14651858.CD003968.pub2.]

Hypnotism as a means of adjusting the perception of pain and attitudes to pain is dealt with elsewhere in this book.

The Doctors

Pain specialists, or pain medicine doctors, are experts at diagnosing the cause of pain and then treating it.

Pain management practitioners come from all fields of medicine. In addition to medical practitioners, a pain management team may often benefit from the input of physiotherapists, clinical psychologists, and occupational therapists, among others.

Anesthesiologists, neurologists, and neurosurgeons most frequently specialize in pain management. Some physiatrists also specialize in pain management.

Pain physicians are often fellowship-trained, board-certified anesthesiologists, neurologists, physiatrists, or psychiatrists. Palliative care doctors are also specialists in pain management.

As the field of pain medicine has grown rapidly, many practitioners have entered the field, some not board-certified. Practitioners lacking a medical fellowship have opted for certification by the American Board of Pain Medicine, which does not require post-graduate medical fellowship training and is not recognized by the American Board of Medical Specialties. That's just politics; your concern is simply: is he (she) any good?

Here's more about these specialists:

Anesthesiologists: These doctors are often the leaders of a team of other specialists and doctors who work together to help manage pain.

The team may include orthopedists (doctors who deal with the prevention or correction of injuries or disorders of the bones and skeletal system), nurse practitioners, physician assistants, physical or rehabilitation therapists, and others.

Neurologists: Doctors who diagnose and treat diseases of the nervous system. Their tools are almost entirely drugs.

Neurosurgeons: Doctors who perform surgery on the nervous system. This is very drastic and final. No use finding a cure later, if that part of the body is gone. Neurosurgeons, in my opinion, are notorious for carrying out unproven and unjustifiable procedures, just for the lure of profits.

Physiatrists: Doctors who specialize in physical medicine, which is a branch of medicine that deals with the treatment, prevention, and diagnosis of disease by physical means, including manipulation, massage, and exercise.

Orthopedic surgeons, who may operate to ablate nerves and remove tissue.

Specific Approaches to Pain Relief

In many senses, it is a question of skilled matching of the type of pain with the patient's experience and capabilities. Types of pain are many and varied, as are its sites, and patients are about as diverse in character and attitude as their numbers.

Certain pains suggest certain types of treatment; certain patients seem to demand a certain approach. There is less "hard science" than proponents might like to believe and perhaps more thoughtful compassion and whimsy than is admitted.

Specific treatments, other than the ones to be found elsewhere in this text, include:

Injections. Local anesthetics, sometimes combined with a corticosteroid, may be injected around nerve roots or into muscles and joints to relieve irritation, swelling, and muscle spasms.

Nerve blocks. If a group of nerves, called a ganglion or plexus, causes pain to a specific organ or body region, injections with local anesthetics may be useful for blocking the pain in that area.

Ablation. This means severing nerves and is a remedy of desperation, when nothing else with suffice. Pulsed radiofrequency modulation and actual severing of nerves may work.

Back Pain. There are many interventional procedures available for pain. Interventional procedures typically used for chronic back pain include epidural steroid injections, facet joint injections, neurolytic blocks, spinal cord stimulators, and intrathecal drug delivery system implants.

A spinal cord stimulator is an implantable medical device that creates electric impulses and applies them near the dorsal surface of the spinal cord, providing a paresthesia ("tingling") sensation that alters the perception of pain by the patient.

An intrathecal pump is used to deliver very small quantities of medications directly to the spinal fluid. This is similar to epidural infusions used in childbirth and postoperatively. The major differences are that it is much more common for the drug to be delivered into the spinal fluid (intrathecal) rather than epidurally, and the pump can be fully implanted under the skin. This approach allows a smaller dose of the drug to be delivered directly to the site of action, with fewer systemic side effects.

Physical Therapy. Physical medicine and rehabilitation (physiatry/physiotherapy) employ diverse physical techniques, such as thermal agents and electrotherapy, as well as therapeutic exercise and behavioral therapy, alone or in tandem with interventional techniques and conventional pharmacotherapy to treat pain.

See also: Understanding Pain Prescriptions, section 2

ACUPUNCTURE

Around 2003, I lived in Sri Lanka, a small island nation in the Indian Ocean (I'd go back at the drop of a hat!)

While I worked there at the Open International University of Complementary Medicines, I saw some remarkable "non-Western" medicine, including acupuncture in operation. It was nothing to see a 5-kilo mass (12 pounds) of tumor removed from near the face with no anesthetic whatever. Just acupuncture.

While doctors in the USA were being indicted and jailed for the "fraud" of acupuncture, the rest of the world was watching sights like this on TV and marveling at how effective it was. Just a few needles placed in just the right places seemed to numb the body of all pain feelings and, if the pain started to re-emerge, a few twizzles on the needles sent the patient back into the state of anesthesia!

No intubation, no anesthetic gases with concomitant danger to life, no chance of cutting the wrong limb off, because the patient is wide-awake conscious!

Not surprisingly then, acupuncture—in the right skilled hands—can tackle milder pain, such as soreness, stiff neck, and arthritis. The only condition for success is that you do have to find the right person, with the requisite skills. There are so many people masquerading as acupuncturists who are badly trained and incompetent, that it is *caveat emptor* (buyer beware).

Nor is it enough just to look for professional certification or approval from a licensing body, because those are notoriously corrupt and really just a trade union, designed to keep outsiders on the outside, while "the boys" carve up the action between themselves.

There are good acupuncturists who wouldn't go near such a professional body!

How Does It Work?

All pain is blocked flow; that's the theory. Get the energies flowing again through the meridians and the pain will dissolve itself.

Ever since the 1970s, when this ancient Chinese tradition debuted in the US, Western researchers have sought to understand the phenomenon of acupuncture. Now proper research is emerging to make it "evidence-based medicine."

A new study of acupuncture, published in the *Archives of Internal Medicine*, one of the most rigorous and detailed studies to date, found that it can ease migraines and arthritis and other forms of chronic pain. [*Arch Intern Med.* 2012; 172(19): 1444-1453. doi: 10.1001/archinternmed.2012.3654.]

That puts paid to the usual dumb criticism: that there is "no proof" it works, or "studies showing it works are of poor quality" (the usual get-out when something unpalatable to narrow-minded orthodox doctors is published).

Financed by the National Institutes of Health and carried out over about half a decade, the new research was a detailed analysis of earlier research that involved data on nearly 18,000 patients and found that acupuncture outperformed placebo and standard treatments when used on people suffering from osteoarthritis, migraines, and chronic back, neck and shoulder pain.

This latest study was relentless in tracking down quality results. The findings were "rigorous," to use the modern term. Hard to argue with, in other words.

You'll get the usual carping critic who claims, "Ah, but it didn't prove it worked for knee pain!" Ignore all such; the results are outstandingly clear: acupuncture is no longer "controversial."

The truth is, acupuncture is among the most widely practiced forms of alternative medicine in the world and is offered by many hospitals, even here in the medically-retarded USA. Most commonly, the treatment is sought by adults looking for relief from chronic pain, though it is also used with growing frequency in children. According to government estimates, about 150,000 children in the United States underwent acupuncture in 2007.

Acupuncture is used as an adjunct treatment or an acceptable alternative to treat an ever-growing list of disorders: addiction, stroke, headache, menstrual cramps, tennis elbow, fibromyalgia, osteoarthritis, low back pain, carpal tunnel syndrome, asthma, infertility, pregnancy problems, dental pain, and side effects from cancer treatment.

One advantage of this type of treatment, admits the US National Institutes of Health, is that the rates of side effects are substantially lower than that of many drugs or other accepted medical procedures used for the same conditions.

Acupuncture is effective for the treatment of chronic pain, said the 2012 study, and is therefore a reasonable referral option. Significant differences between true and sham acupuncture indicate that acupuncture is more than a placebo.

However, the authors noted the differences were not spectacular, suggesting that the wise course of action was to include acupuncture, if you are inclined to use it, along with other pain-modifying techniques listed in this book. Do not rely on acupuncture alone.

I repeat what I said earlier—I have seen it produce *amazing* results. So it's your call!

Musculoskeletal Points

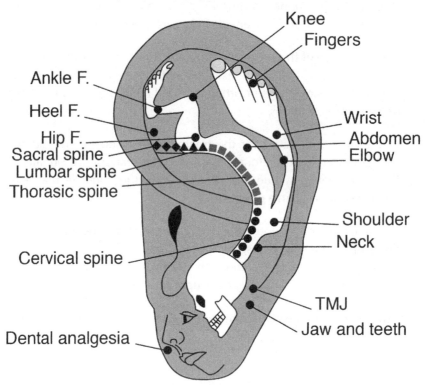

This schematic representation of the human body on the outer ear is a distortion of the shape, as you can see.

But the layout bears a remarkable resemblance to an upside down replication of our anatomy. Points can be stimulated by needles or studs, or even just finger pressure.

Some points are great for relieving pain. If the pain recurs or is chronic, you can wear a stud in the appropriate point. You then stimulate it by pressing or twiddling the stud whever you feel uncomfortable.

There are, of course, numerous other points which can be used for addictions and other kinds of pathology. This diagram is for illustrative purposes only, not instructional.

EAR ACUPUNCTURE

Nogier's Auriculo-Acupuncture Method

There is another variant of acupuncture you may not have heard of. It rests on the fact that most acupuncture points are replicated on the outer ear (the pinna) and therefore is called auriculo-acupuncture.

Historically, the Chinese, Arabs, Romanies, Hindus, and some Europeans advocated needling a point on the ear lobe to remedy eye deficiencies. Even today, some European doctors recommend the insertion of a gold or silver earring to stimulate this spot continuously in cases of eye deficiency.

An ancient Indian text, the *Suchi Veda* (which translated means "Science of Needle Piercing") gives detailed techniques and points for needling the ears. It is interesting that the Arabs should use the ear mainly for the treatment of low back pain and kidney trouble, when it is known that the ear is seen by the Chinese as the outward "flowering" of the kidneys.

Ear acupuncture was revived in modern times by the French doctor, Paul Nogier, and published in 1951. Apparently (so the story goes), he sometimes saw patients who had had cauterization of points on the ear and who claimed to have been relieved of their sciatica as a result of this treatment.

After several years of experimentation, Nogier revived auriculo-acupuncture and established a map of the acupuncture points on the outer ear (see diagram). Each point generally named for its related anatomy, e.g., lung, heart, knee, elbow, brain etc.

It's usually pointed out that these points fairly closely resemble the image of an inverted homunculus or fetus. That might be fancy or maybe is a strong clue to why this works as it does. Auriculo-therapy has even been important back into China, where it has sparked a wave of research into the apparent embryonic connections.

Currently, auriculo-acupuncture is much used for anesthesia, weight loss, and addictions, particularly smoking. I have a good friend who decided to test the "dental anesthesia" point by squeezing it hard and she reported to me it worked very well, allowing the dentist to drill her tooth without an injection of local.

To be really *sure* it was working, she relaxed her pressure during the procedure, squealed with pain and rapidly re-asserted her firm grip on that part of the ear!

Diagnosis can be done by finding tender or painful points. These are then treated with pressure (squeezing), needles and studs, laser, or even electrical stimulation.

Devices

P-Stim. The P-Stim (Biegler GmbH, Mauerbach, Austria) is a portable auricular electro-acupuncture stimulation device used for the treatment of pain. Compared to conventional acupuncture, it has the advantage of continuous auricular stimulation for up to four days.

You can take a crack at self-treatment using the auriculo-acupuncture approach. There are several simple electrical devices on the market, like the Medicomat-15, which is sold on Amazon and costs $160 at the time of writing. [*Acupunct Med.* 2009; 27: 187-188. doi:10.1136/aim.2009.001388

HOMOTOXICOLOGY

For this pain treatment modality, I am going to have to teach you a whole new medical paradigm. I already explained in the introduction that it's not in my nature to just throw you tidbits. I'd rather play my full role as educator and teach you what you need to know to progress through life safely and with the skills and knowledge to at least defend yourself, even if you don't aspire to therapeutic abilities.

You should find it an interesting journey and you can always look further into things, if you become captivated by the model. Once again, it goes well beyond just treating the symptom: pain relief. It's about solving problems and restoring health.

I sometimes call this treatment modality "deep tissue cleansing" because that comes closer than anything to describing what's actually going in. I'm talking about eliminating toxins from the body and putting a stop to the negative effects they have, unless dealt with properly and terminatedly.

I'm talking now about homotoxicology; "homo-" (the same) in this sense means "own toxins." Despite its clumsy name, homotoxicology is a wonderful natural healing science. It is a therapeutic branch that enables deep cleansing of the body tissues, removing old toxins, disease processes and degenerative debris, leaving the fluids clean, fresh, and able to function as intended.

Based on homeopathy, but not quite the same thing, homotoxicology is the brain child of German doctor Hans-Heinrich Reckeweg (1905-1985). Knowing homeopathy and drawing on a vast knowledge of herbal lore and medicines, he compounded a store of remedies which trod a line between folk medicine and basic plant pharmacology. In the course of time, it has proved itself so well that tens of thousands of German doctors use it in daily practice, although it is less well-known in the rest of the world.

It has been also called the German system of homeopathy, though this is slightly comical, since the original, classical system of homeopathy was also invented by a German, Samuel Hahnemann. It's also sometimes known as complex homeopathy, not because it is complicated, but because it uses mixtures or complexes.

Another term used for this approach to healing is *bioregulatory* medicine; the Germans love these clunky, compounded words; it's how their language works.

The Matrix in Health and Disease

Whereas so much molecular medicine is aimed at the cell, as if it were the sole seat of disease, Dr. Alfred Pischinger, then professor of Histology and Embryology in Vienna, saw with great insight that the extracellular fluids were the key to health. These fluids, which Pischinger called the "matrix," or ground regulation system, support everything else, bringing nutrition, oxygen, hormone messengers, and other vital substances to the tissues and removing excretion products, toxins, and the residue of old diseases.

Cells may be important but are not a separate entity because they cannot exist without being nurtured in this matrix. In this sense, modern medicine has blinded itself and somehow ignores the obvious role of the support mechanisms.

Reckeweg pursued Pischinger's matrix model and devised ways to use natural substances to support, clean, and revitalize the extracellular matrix. That's what homotoxicology does. Most of the classic homeopathic remedies are still there, though used slightly differently.

The point is that pain relief is far more thorough and permanent if the whole landscape of the body is cleaned up. Then the pain nerves have nothing to complain about and fall silent!

I have reproduced a schematic diagram of the matrix here. I hope it sheds some light.

Pischinger's matrix

It shows the matrix being fed by blood from the heart and drained away by venous blood and lymphatic drainage (doctors tend to forget this aspect of tissue hygiene). The connective tissue cells are floating in the extracellular fluid. The whole is supplied by the nervous system, which helps regulate it. But many chemical messengers also control this matrix: hormones, of course. Also cytokines (literally means "cell motivators").

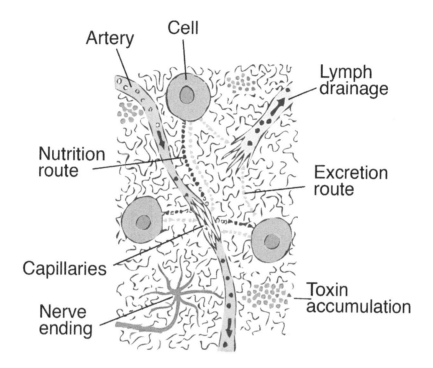

Cleansing the Matrix

So, if we can help this internal transport system, and find ways to detox it, so that it is running sweetly, we can work wonders for health and reduce or eliminate symptoms due to the matrix becoming burdened with toxins.

To do that, we use remedy mixtures, compounded with the end in mind. Reckeweg made formulas that would support the liver and kidneys, that would work for flu, diabetes, and women's problems, stimulate metabolism, tone up the immune system, retard tumors, repair inflammation, act as painkillers, and so on. In other words, these are function-based medicines.

The remedies are homeopathically diluted but not so much. We rarely see the large dilutions of classical homeopathy, in which none of the original substance is present (something that drives ignorant doctors and scientists wild!)

Reckeweg's original company was called HEEL (stands for *herba est ex luce*: Latin for "plants are from light"). Reckeweg is long deceased but HEEL is still there in Baden-Baden, Germany. I mention it because you can find one of Reckeweg's most famous formulas in almost any health store in Europe and the USA—even in Whole Foods, USA—it's called Traumeel and, as you might guess, it's for trauma or injury. See? You already knew something about this! (Most of HEELs remedies end in "eel.")

Having said that, I must now say there are many other fine companies in this space, too, and they manufacture superb products that are among the most effective and yet gentle remedies that I know. Specifically, I will mention Guna (Italy), Deseret Biologicals (Utah), HEEL-BHI (Biological Homeopathic Industries), Albuquerque (started here by Reckeweg after retirement but not related, commercially, to the Baden-Baden company), and Pascoe (Friedrich H. Pascoe (1867-1930).

Chords

As well as mixtures of remedies, some formulas are a single remedy in a mixtures of potencies (called a "chord," after the musical term for several notes sounding at once).

There are key advantages to using potency chords:

- Layers of action, so going deeper
- Fewer initial aggravations than classical dosing
- Doses can be repeated
- Broader spectrum of effect
- No problems selecting the appropriate potency
- No problems in assessing the duration or spectrum of action
- Mixing high and low potencies produces an effect that lies somewhere in between: rapid onset (low potency) and long-lasting action (high potency)
- Faster action
- Potency stages retain their own effects

Then there are homaccords, which are mixtures of chords and multiple remedies (you don't need to memorize this; there's no exam!)

So, for example HEEL's Nux Vomica Homaccord (*nux vom* is a classic detox substance, going back to the time of Hildegard of Bingen). This particular preparation contains:

Colocynthis 3X (0.15ml)
Colocynthis 10X (0.15ml)
Colocynthis 30X (0.15ml)
Colocynthis 200X (0.15ml)
Lycopodium clavatum 3X (0.15ml)
Lycopodium clavatum 10X (0.15ml)
Lycopodium clavatum 30X (0.15ml)
Lycopodium clavatum 200X (0.15ml)
Lycopodium clavatum 1000X (0.15ml)
Bryonia alba 3X (0.1ml)
Bryonia alba 6X (0.1ml)
Bryonia alba 10X (0.1ml)
Bryonia alba 15X (0.1ml)
Bryonia alba 30X (0.1ml)
Bryonia alba 200X (0.1ml)
Bryonia alba 1000X (0.1ml)
Nux vomica 3X (0.1ml)
Nux vomica 10X (0.1ml)
Nux vomica 15X (0.1ml)
Nux vomica 30X (0.1ml)
Nux vomica 200X (0.1ml)
Nux vomica 1000X (0.1ml)

See page 60 for explanation of the potencies.

Dosing Regimen

Depending on the exact remedy, these preparations can come as tablets, creams and ointments, or glass ampoules. The latter are made for IV administration but there's a trick that enables you to take the remedy without needing a doctor or nurse to give you an IV:

Dissolve one ampoule in a bottle of spring water (preferably glass bottled, so no BPA, phthalates, etc.) Sip it throughout the day (no rush!) Then skip two days.

Repeat. In other words, one day on and two days off. If you are taking two remedies at once, A and B, you go:

- Day 1: A
- Day 2: B
- Day 3: nil
- Day 4: A
- Day 5: B
- Day 6: nil, and so on…

Traumeel and other remedies work best from the ampoules. But creams and tablets are almost as good. Dose as prescribed.

Homeopathic Trials

Homotoxicology works well for pain and inflammatory conditions, including rheumatoid arthritis, fibromyalgia, bursitis, back pain, acute sprain, sports injuries, migraines, and headaches.

There have been a number of trials of Traumeel, including for its efficacy in the treatment of sprained ankles. In a reasonably large randomized, blinded, and controlled multi-center study published in 2012, 449 physically active men and women (age 18-40) with a mild to moderate sprain of the ankle (grade 1 and 2) were treated. They were administered with Traumeel ointment (n=152), Traumeel gel (n=150) or diclofenac gel (n=147).

There was little difference in the results between the three medications, in terms of reducing symptoms of inflammation, accelerating recovery, and improving mobility. But of course Traumeel is far less dangerous than NSAIDs (see page 25). It's also far cheaper.

While continued research and development is ongoing to broaden the clinical evidence of Traumeel in acute musculoskeletal injury and to further establish its benefits, current information suggests that Traumeel may be considered as an anti-inflammatory agent that is at least as effective and appears to be better tolerated than NSAIDs. [De Vega CG, et al. A randomized, controlled, multicentre study on the effectiveness of Traumeel (ointment and gel) in terms of pain reduction and functional improvement compared with diclofenac gel in acute ankle sprain. Abstract EULAR12-4940 presented at the European League Against Rheumatism (EULAR) Congress, Berlin, Germany, June 6-9, 2012.]

This same medicine was also used in the treatment of traumatic hemarthrosis (joint swollen with blood) and was shown to significantly reduce healing time, as compared to a placebo. Objective measurements of joint swelling and movement and evaluation of the synovial fluid at injury were assessed.

Other Pain Control Preparations

There are numerous choices for pain control in this class of medications. Here are just some examples from the HEEL practitioner manual.

Ankylosing spondylitis	*Traumeel, Zeel*
Arthritis	*Zeel*
Back pain, lumbago, sciatica	*Colocynthis Homaccord*
Gall bladder	*Chelidonium-Homaccord*
Colitis	*Podophyllum comp*
Dislocations and sprains	*Traumeel*
Gout	*Lithiumeel*
Colic	*Spascupreel*
Endometriosis, dysmenoorhea	*Gynaäcoheel*
Irritable bowel, with pains	*Nux vomica-Homaccord*
Kidney stones	*Atropinum compositum*
Migraine	*Psorinoheel*
Muscular rheumatism, fibrositis	*Colocynthis-Homaccord and Rhododendronneel*
Neuralgia	*Colocynthis-Homaccord and Spigelia comp.*
Pancreatitis	*Momorcordia comp.*
Prostatitis	*Sabal-HomaccordomaccordHo*
Shingles	*Ranunculus-Homaccord*
Snake bite	*Arnica-Heel*
Sports injuries, dislocations	*Traumeel*
TMJ syndrome	*Zeel or Traumeel*
Trigeminal neuralgia	*Spigelon*

A Completely Novel Approach To Pain

I have hinted all the way through this book that improving overall health issues has great benefit for reducing or eliminating pain. After all, pain means something is wrong. It should not be suppressed with analgesics but some attempt needs to be made to get to the cause of the problem and eradicate it.

There are many ways to use homotoxicology to improve health, such as clearing old vaccination and childhood diseases (the effect may be lingering in the matrix fluid); stimulating detox organs, such as liver and kidneys; rejuvenating tissues, with things like lively placenta tissue; improving blood flow and cardiac performance; and what we call "drainage," which is to say getting the matrix circulation flowing properly, as per the diagram above.

We can also energize tissues by boosting what is called the Kreb's cycle. This is the pathway where glucose is metabolized, creating adenosine triphosphate (ATP) molecules, which are our principal source of cellular energy in the mitochondria. Basically, the Kreb's cycle is a series of eight enzyme reactions, which take place sequentially.

Any disruption in the cycle stops the process. The therapeutic idea behind the "bio-catalyst" products is to administer the citric acid cycle intermediates in a series of steps, until all the intermediates have been taken. If there is a particularly strong reaction at any one of the steps, attention can be focused on that intermediate, which can be given as part of the therapy program.

Research has shown that the addition of specific enzyme substances will induce the enzymes into action. This way, if the citric acid cycle is disrupted at any point, adding the intermediate at that point will cause the cycle to pick up again. ATP will be produced and energy will be available to the body for reactions and to ward off disease. Overall health will pick up.

HEEL have prepared a series of homeopathic "boosters" for each stage of this cycle plus two extras (boxes of 10). We call them the intermediate catalysts, though the full name is "bio-catalysts of the citric acid cycle." The individual catalyst names are of no importance to you. Just remember the boxed set! Hopefully, if you are working with someone skilled in this therapy, he or she will be very familiar with them anyway.

This approach is one of the great boosts against the slowing-down process of aging.

Some Conditions That Can Benefit from Intermediate Catalyst Therapy

- Paresis, neuralgia, toxic neuritis, vegetative dystonia, migraine
- Eczema ("neurodermitis"), itching (including pruritus vulvae), psoriasis, vitiligo, pemphigus, scleroderma
- Bronchial asthma
- Gastric and duodenal ulcer, hepatosis, cirrhosis of the liver and injurious hepatic disorders, pancreopathy
- Kidney disease, e.g., nephrosis and chronic nephritis
- Myocardial impairment, angina pectoris, treatment subsequent to myocardial infarction, arteriosclerosis, cerebral sclerosis
- Hormone dysfunction and dysregulation of endocrine glands, e.g., diabetes mellitus, over- and under-active thyroid
- Pre-cancerous and de-differentiation phases (previously: neoplasm phases) within any tissue whatsoever
- During and ensuing X-ray and radioactive exposure (several enzymes, e.g., maleate dehydrogenase, are sensitive to radiation)
- Blood manufacturing disorders: thrombocytopenia, leucopenia

Depending on local laws in your country, you may be able to prescribe homotoxicology for yourself. Very many of Reckeweg's remedies are available over the counter and by mail order. Surprisingly, Traumeel is the one you may have most trouble with, because it contains *Aconite* (monkshood) which is highly toxic, yet only diluted to the 3rd potency (3X). It's OK in the USA though.

Also—don't forget all of these remedies—and there are hundreds—can be used with the biopuncture method (page 63).

Biographical note: I was on the advisory board for Homotoxicology UK for many years and on the speaker list for HEEL, Baden-Baden.

Homeopathic First Aid

BACH'S RESCUE REMEDY

It would be a big mistake not to mention Bach's so-called "Rescue Remedy". It's not for pain, as such, but for shock, trauma, injury and anything which shakes a person up temporarily.

It's a homeopathic preparation of five flower remedies: Impatiens, Star of Bethlehem, Cherry Plum, Rock Rose and Clematis.

This mix was created by Dr. Edward Bach to deal with emergencies and crises – the moments when there is no time to make a proper individual selection of remedies.

The Rescue Remedy is designed to help deal with immediate problems. If you are working through an underlying problem – or if you seem to need rescuing every day – you will find a longer-term solution by selecting a personal blend of remedies.

Put 10 drops into a tumbler of water and sip it over an hour or two. Repeat if needed. You can also dab drops behind your ear, on the forehead or on the wrists, to good effect.

More information at the Bach Remedies website:
www.BachFlower.com

CALENDULA CREAM

Calendula officianalis (Marigold) is a much-loved remedy. It's great for painful skin conditions, such as cuts, scratches, scuffs, burns, scalds, too much sun, or fiery eczema. You should always have a tube of this handy.

For minor burns, immediately run cool water on the burn for several minutes and dry. Then apply plentiful Calendula Cream to the affected area 3 - 4 times a day or as needed.

For cuts, scrapes and shallow wounds, first cleanse the area with mild soap, rinse and dry, before applying the cream.

You can also get sprays and balm. Incidentally, Calendula is listed in the US Homeopathic Pharmacopeia.

The Meaning Of Homeopthic Potencies

It is important to understand the following characteristics of how homeopathic "nanopharmacy" medicines are made.

1. Most homeopathic medicines are made by diluting a medicinal substance in a double-distilled water. It should be noted that physicists who study the properties of water commonly acknowledge that water has many mysterious properties. Because homeopaths use a double-distilled water, it is highly purified, enabling the medicinal sub-

stance to solely infiltrate the water. The medicinal solution is usually preserved in an 87% water/alcohol solution.

2. Each substance is diluted, most commonly, 1 part of the original medicinal agent to 9 or 99 parts double-distilled water. This is the C series (c for 100). The mixture is then vigorously stirred or shaken. The solution is then diluted again 1:9 or 1:99 and vigorously stirred. This process of diluting and stirring is repeated 3, 6, 12, 30, 200, 1,000, or even 1,000,000 times.

3. Another common sequence is the 1 in 10 or D (decimal series), sometimes known as the X series (Roman numeral X).

4. It is inaccurate to say that homeopathic medicines are just extremely diluted; they are extremely "potentized." Potentization refers to the specific process of sequential dilution with vigorous stirring. The theory is that each consecutive dilution in conjunction with the process of shaking/stirring infiltrates the new double-distilled water and imprints upon it the fractal form of the original substance used (fractal refers to the specific consecutively smaller pattern or form within a larger pattern).

BIOPUNCTURE

Biopuncture therapy, developed by my friend Jan Kersschot in Belgium, is gaining international recognition. It is useful for pain.

It's similar to neural therapy but definitely a separate modality. Instead of using anesthetics or toxins (lidocaine, bee venom, etc.), it uses gentle homeopathic remedies. The idea is to inject the remedy superficially, into skin or muscles, close to the organ or region of dysfunction.

Products commonly used are, for example, arnica, echinacea, nux vomica and chamomile. Arnica is used for muscle pain, nux vomica is injected for digestive problems, and echinacea is used to increase the natural defense system of the body.

Biopuncturists always inject cocktails of natural products. Lymphomyosot is used for lymphatic drainage, Traumeel for inflammations and sports injuries, Spascupreel for muscular cramps, and so on. This range of products are from HEEL (Baden-Baden), for which Jan is an agent. I myself am a champion of these remedies.

Most of the ampoules used for injection are made in Germany and are held to very strict quality control regulations. Clinical studies on thousands of patients have confirmed the safety of ampoules such as Traumeel.

But other remedies from Guna (Italy), Deseret Biologicals (Utah), etc., where appropriate for injection, may be used instead.

The treatment is completely safe, because the ampoules contain high concentrations of active substances. As a result, toxic side effects are very unlikely.

Biopuncture therapy is done with remedies that are not so extremely dilute as classical homeopathy, so we call them ultra-low doses.

The target effect varies widely but almost all remedies are intended to act on the intercellular fluid matrix and will, in time, remove toxins and metabolites that may be causing pain and inflammation.

The reaction of your body may be, for example, better local blood circulation, tissue repair, relaxation of muscles, or local detoxification. During the reparation of tissue, your body is even more vulnerable and it is a good idea at this stage not to overuse the part that is treated because it is still in the process of repair.

In addition, organs can be stimulated and healed; old diseases expelled; and tissues toned and invigorated, so that self-healing takes place. These ultra-low doses "wake up" mechanisms that are available anyway. So, the healing effect comes from "inside" your body—not from the therapeutic products themselves.

How can such a small dose influence your body and stimulate healing? Scientists don't have the final proof yet, but they postulate that these injections are working through the stimulation of the body's natural defense systems, such as the immune system and detox pathways.

Recent research on biopuncture has given new insight into how these products seem to do the job. For example, scientific investigation has illustrated that Traumeel indeed works via the immune system. In June 2004, an article was published in an important medical journal, *Clinical & Developmental Immunology*, which is a highly respected journal in conventional medicine. Your physician will be surprised to hear that the mechanisms of action of Traumeel include both inhibition of IL-1ß and inhibition of TNF-alpha secretion.

If your doctor really wants to know more about this study or is interested in other clinical studies on biopuncture, he or she can find more information in the textbooks on biopuncture.

Procedure

Most people are surprised at how easily and quickly these injections are given. In fact, these injections cannot be compared to the "usual" injections given in conventional medicine. They are not as painful as an injection in, for example, a hospital because the needle used is exceptionally fine and the quantity injected is very small. Most of them are given into or just under the skin, others are given into specific muscle points or into your ligaments (= bands that hold bones together).

The biopuncturist doesn't give the injections arbitrarily, but they are administered in carefully chosen spots. The place where the practitioner injects you is as important as the product itself and is different for each patient.

Usually you will receive multiple injections at a site. For example, if your doctor wants to work on your liver, he or she will give about seven little injections under the skin on your belly, just under the rib margin on the right side.

When you have pain in your elbow, your physician will look for several painful spots in your arm muscles or elbow ligaments, and inject each of them in one session. In such a case, you may receive anything from three to ten small injections in your elbow, neck or arm.

It's a slow, gentle therapy, not a one-shot blast. But it is highly effective and has far greater benefits than merely the relief of pain. It is truly a healing modality.

If you have had problems for several months or even years, your biopuncturist needs to work on different layers. If it is a complicated case, he (or she) must also look for deeper causes of your complaints and work on these. This may be the case when treating, for example, headaches or migraine: sometimes your hormonal system has to be regulated; or you need a detoxification ("cleaning" of the body) first. As a result, you may need several sessions to feel the results of the treatment.

Detoxing

That's a word that's bandied around a lot these days. In biopuncture, detoxing removes tissue and fluid contaminants that may be present in organs, tissues, lymphatics, and extracellular fluid.

The modality, called homotoxicology (dealing with "own toxins") is a whole discipline in itself and beyond the range of this book on pain therapies.

In addition to homotoxins, there is the question of iatrogenic toxins (vaccinations feature a lot), drugs (which are alien chemicals), smoking, environmental pollution, and many other exposures to undesirable and toxic substances.

Bad nutrition with today's synthetic diets can also lay in large numbers of toxins.

These toxins can block your defense system. So you will find a good biopuncturist working on eliminating toxins. To do that he or she uses what are called "drainage remedies." Drainage, or elimination of toxins, is via the liver, gut, kidneys, lungs, and skin. It is like taking the leaves out of the gutter.

The body is very adept at it but cannot cope if the toxin burden is too high and will need help from drainage remedies such as lymphomyosot, a remedy considered very important in biopuncture.

The down side of such an approach is that old symptoms (which have been suppressed earlier on) may come to the surface again. But that is sometimes part of the healing strategy of the body. There is an old law that says healing comes from the inside out and goes backwards through time (so if you arthritis was once asthma, the asthma will re-appear when the arthritis fades). It's striking but one of the well-known phenomena of holistic healing.

Pain Specifically

Neck pain and back pain respond well to biopuncture, but one can also treat ankle sprains, pain in the shoulder, and Achilles tendonitis using these natural injections. Biopuncture is also very successful in treating tennis elbow and golf elbow.

However, biopuncture is not just used for pain problems, osteoarthritis or sports injuries. An area of treatment worth noting is that of allergies and inflammations. For example, one can treat asthma, eczema and hay fever. And even patients with bronchitis, cystitis and sinusitis can be treated with this technique. When a physician is experienced in the technique, he or she can also treat you for migraine, tension headache, sciatica, and so on.

Biopuncture is an interesting healing technique for those patients who want to avoid surgery (for example, for sciatica or sinusitis). In some patients it may be advantageous to combine the conventional approach with biopuncture. Each case should be taken into account individually, of course.

For more information, visit Jan Kersschot's website: www.kersschot. com

See also: Homotoxicology

NEURAL THERAPY

Neural therapy is a method of treating pain and other illnesses caused by disturbances of the body's electrophysiology. These electrical disturbances, called "interference fields," are manifestations of cell membrane instability and typically trigger abnormal autonomic nervous system responses. Interference fields may be found in scars, autonomic ganglia, teeth and jaw, internal organs, or other locations where local tissue irritation exists.

Neural therapy was developed in Germany, beginning in the 1920s, by two German physician-dentist brothers, Walter and Ferdinand Huneke. They found by serendipity that procaine—a local anesthetic—when injected into certain spots such as scars, can relieve pain in areas nowhere near the place of injection!

They also found that the pain relief lasts much longer than would be expected from the anesthetic effect alone.

A considerable body of scientific research supports its basic principles; unfortunately, almost all of the literature is published in German and has never been translated into English. Texts in English are now becoming more readily available.

What Characterizes Interference Fields?

Interference fields have lower (or higher) electrical potentials than surrounding tissues. Currents flow from areas of higher voltage to areas of lower voltage and seem to send confusing signals to the body's nervous system. The body sometimes reacts in inappropriate ways, resulting in altered autonomic nervous system tone, chronic pain, and/or dysfunction.

Interference fields can be found almost anywhere in the body and are often far from the part of the body experiencing symptoms. For example, an old appendix scar might cause migraine headache, or a wisdom tooth extraction scar may cause chronic low-back pain. For the most part, these relationships are totally unpredictable and interference fields must be searched for everywhere in the body.

The traditional way of finding these fields is by taking a careful history of the patient's problem to look for an injury, operation, or illness in the months or years preceding the onset of symptoms. Presumably, part of the body's response to the injury or illness was a local "alarm reaction" involving the autonomic nervous system. The autonomic nervous system changes circulation to a body part when an emergency affects that area of the body. Interference fields seem to develop when the autonomic nervous system control does not return to normal after the emergency.

2. Palpate possible trouble spots while testing the patient's muscle strength.

Another way of finding interference fields is by making use of the body's electromagnetic field. The electromagnetic field of the body depends on the generation of electricity by healthy tissue. If tissue is not receiving adequate circulation, as in an interference field, it will be less vigorous and not have as strong an electromagnetic field over it.

The interference field can be "boosted" temporarily by another person (usually the physician), touching the spot with his or her hand. When this occurs, there is a generalized inhibition of all the patient's muscles. Thus, the physician can search for interference fields by touching possible spots while testing the patient's muscle strength.

What conditions are likely to be caused by an interference field?

Any symptom related to bodily functions controlled by the autonomic nervous system, such as palpitations, brochospasm, indigestion, constipation, sexual dysfunction, dysmenorrhea, or even cold hands or feet may be partially or totally caused by an interference field.

Chronic pain—especially migraine—often has an autonomic component, such as nausea or sweating. An interference field may also be suspected if sciatica or any other leg pain is accompanied by coldness or change in skin color.

How does neural therapy treat interference fields?

If an interference field is found, it can be easily treated by injecting it with a local anesthetic, such as lidocaine. The effect of injecting interference fields is immediate. There is sometimes sudden relief of symptoms—a "lightning reaction"— but any response typically will occur within the first few days.

In recent years, a non-injection therapy has been developed that seems to work as well as the -caine anesthetics. A proprietary electrical device called a Tenscam® is held approximately 18 inches from the body and directed at the interference field for a minute or two.

More often than not, response to treatment of an interference field is temporary, sometimes lasting even less than a day. However, even a very short response is encouraging and indicates that treatment should be attempted again. Each time an interference field is treated, there should be a longer response. Treatment is then repeated until it is no longer required.

How safe is neural therapy?

Neural therapy is a remarkably safe medical treatment. The most commonly used anesthetics (procaine and lidocaine) rarely cause allergic reactions. Allergic reactions to these anesthetics in the past seem to have been caused by preservatives such as methylparaben. These preservatives are no longer used by most physicians practicing neural therapy.

Occasionally, patients will feel faint for a few minutes after neural therapy injections. This may be caused by "needle fright" or by a short-lasting lowering of the blood pressure caused by the -caine anesthetic itself. Puncture of an internal organ is a theoretical possibility with certain injections. Because the needles used are of small caliber, this is rarely (if ever) of any consequence. The one exception is the lung which, if punctured, may cause a pneumothorax. For this reason, special care must be taken with any deep injection into the chest wall or near the lungs. Another area of injection that carries a slight risk is the head and neck. Injection of a large volume of anesthetic into an artery could precipitate a seizure. To avoid this, injections in the head and neck are always performed slowly, drawing back on the syringe from time to time to make sure the needle has not penetrated an artery.

What conditions may prevent successful treatment?

- **Medications.** The most common reason for poor response to neural therapy treatment is the presence of medication. Any drug with a prefix of "anti-" tends to block the autonomic nervous system, e.g., antibiotics, anti-inflammatories, antidepressants, and antihypertensives. Illicit drugs will block it as well.

- **Poor nutrition.** Inadequate nutrition is much more common than most people realize. Mineral and vitamin deficiencies must be corrected or interference fields will either recur or the response to treatment will not increase with time.

- **Toxins. Drugs, tobacco and alcohol** may be considered toxins and can cause a poor response to neural therapy. Environmental toxins such as organic solvents, herbicides, and fungicides also affect some people. The metals in dental amalgam fillings, especially mercury, poison the autonomic nervous system and may defeat neural therapy.

When and where did neural therapy originate?

Neural therapy is a remarkably safe and simple method of treating many medical problems and is taught in German medical schools. Only in recent years have some in the English-speaking world of medicine become aware of neural therapy.

Types of Pain That Will Respond

- Acute or chronic joint pain (segmental therapy and all scars)
- Post-herpetic neuralgia (Herpes zoster in the chronic stage, not in the acute stage)
- Post 3rd-degree burn pain (segmental therapy)
- Fibromyalgia (injections over the areas of tenderness, all scars, adrenals, thyroid)
- Kidney failure (segmental therapy over the kidney area twice a week)
- Depression and chronic fatigue (segmental therapy to scars, skull, thyroid, and adrenal area)
- Facial pain, trigeminal neuralgia and TMJ pain
- Premature aging and hormonal imbalances (same treatment as 6.)

Treatment schedule: Any condition may respond to a single treatment or may require a series of injections. These should be given initially twice a week, later once a week. If there is no sign of improvement after four treatments, I discontinue this modality.

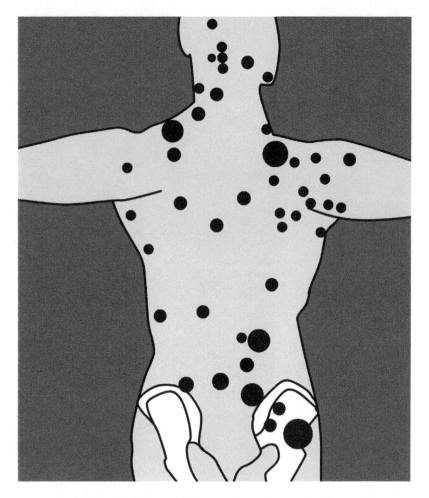

All over the body, notably in muscles and connective tissues, there lurk unpleasant tension points that can cause pain. We call them "trigger points" because they trigger pain.

Some occur at the same site in pretty well everyone. Others are unique to the individual. Practitioners of this kind of therapy are skilled at knowing where trigger points lie and in deducing which one is the likely culprit.

Often the trigger point is some way away from where the actual pain is perceived.

In any case, guessing wrong isn't a big deal. The practitioner chooses a different one and anesthetizes that. Just make sure you are pain-free before leaving the clinic or office and you'll do fine.

TRIGGER POINTS

Similar, again, to neural therapy, is the concept of pain "trigger points" or myofascial trigger points. *Myo-* means muscle and *fascia* is just the scientific name for fibrous sheets associated with muscle (the silvery-white stuff you cut off a good steak!)

We'll stick to the term "trigger points."

It's a pain model that was developed by J. H. Kellgren at University College Hospital, London, in the 1930s and then, independently, by Michael Gutstein in Berlin and Michael Kelly in Australia. The latter two workers continued to publish into the 1950s and 1960s. Kellgren conducted experiments in which he injected hypertonic saline into healthy volunteers and showed that this gave rise to zones of distant or referred extremity pain.

As with the interference fields of neural therapy, the actual hot spot may be far away from where the pain is felt.

Studies estimate that in 75–95% of cases, myofascial pain is a primary cause of regional pain. Myofascial pain is associated with muscle tenderness that arises from trigger points, which are focal points of tenderness, a few millimeters in diameter, found at multiple sites in a muscle and the fascia of muscle tissue.

While nearly everyone has experienced muscle tension pain, the discomfort associated with myofascial pain syndrome persists or worsens. Treatment options for myofascial pain syndrome include physical therapy and trigger point injections. Pain medications and relaxation techniques also can help.

Stress and anxiety caused by the painful condition tends to make it worse.

What Is a Trigger Point?

The term "trigger point" was coined in 1942 by Dr. Janet Travell to describe a clinical finding with the following characteristics:

Pain related to a discrete, irritable point in skeletal muscle or fascia, not caused by acute local trauma, inflammation, degeneration, neoplasm, or infection (in other words, no obvious existing cause).

The painful point can be felt as a nodule or band in the muscle and a twitch response can be elicited on stimulation of the trigger point.

Palpation of the trigger point reproduces the patient's complaint of pain and the pain radiates in a distribution typical of the specific muscle harboring the trigger point.

The pain cannot be explained by findings on neurological examination

Practitioners do not necessarily agree on what constitutes a trigger point. In general, it is accepted that compression of a trigger point may elicit local tenderness, referred pain, or local twitch response (not the same as a muscle spasm).

In a June 2000 review, Chang-Zern Hong correlates some trigger points to acupuncture "ah shi" ("Oh Yes!") points, based on a 1977 paper by Melzack et al. Peter Dorsher remarks on a strong correlation between the locations of trigger points and classical acupuncture points. Apparently 92% of the 255 recognized trigger points correspond to acupuncture points, including 79.5% with similar pain indications.

Diagnosis of Trigger Points

Trigger points are diagnosed by examining signs, symptoms, and pain patterns, and by manual palpation.

Signs and symptoms of myofascial pain syndrome may include deep, aching pain in a muscle, pain that persists or worsens and a tender knot may be felt in a muscle. There may be difficulty sleeping, due to pain.

Usually on examination, there is a taut band or hard nodules that can be felt in the muscles containing the trigger point. Often a twitch response can be felt in the muscle by running your finger perpendicular to the muscle's direction; this twitch response often activates the "all or nothing" response in a muscle that causes it to contract.

Pressing on an affected muscle can often refer pain, meaning the pain is felt elsewhere. Clusters of trigger points are not uncommon in some of the larger muscles, such as the gluteus group in the buttocks.

Sometimes a trigger point feels hot and practitioners can sense that.

Treatment

The trigger point may be subdued by injection of a local anesthetic such as procaine hydrochloride (without adrenalin added), injections without anesthetics (dry needling), and injections of saline, steroids, and even botulinum toxin.

Among physicians, many specialists are well versed in trigger point diagnosis and therapy. These include physiatrists (physicians specializing in physical medicine and rehabilitation), family medicine, and orthopedics. Osteopathic as well as chiropractic schools also include trigger points in their training. Other health professionals, such as athletic trainers, occupational therapists, physiotherapists, acupuncturists, massage therapists, and structural integrators are also aware of these ideas and many of them make use of trigger points in their clinical work as well.

Patients can gently massage their own trigger points.

Controversy

Naturally, there is some dispute about this whole model. But studies using magnetic resonance images and showing abnormalities matching so-called trigger points suggest that the phenomenon is very real. Results were all consistent with the concept that taut muscle fibers are the cause, in which stiffness may be 50% greater than that of the surrounding muscle tissue.

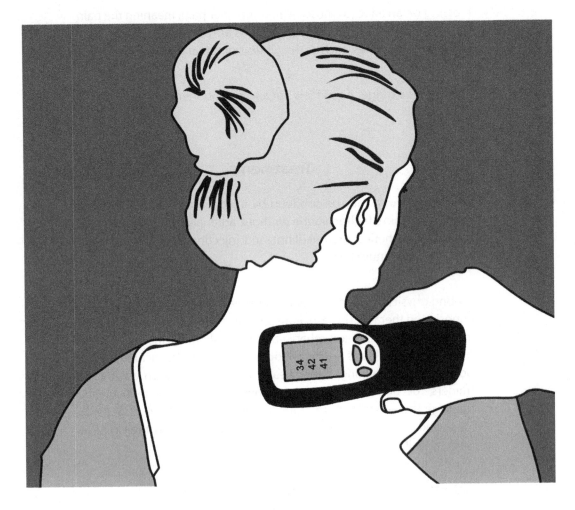

This device is so simple to use, anyone can benefit from it. It's virtually impossible to do it "wrong". The device has smart sensors and so can detect changes in the body and respond with fresh input, without the user having much experience in use.

The first time I used a SCENAR I barely knew how to turn it on. Yet it relieved a friend's arthritis pain for months, after just one treatment!

On the other hand, if you are a professional health practitioner, this is the one must-have device that will enable you to heal a wide range of pathology in a very short time. Families with such a device will get a lot of new visitors, who just happen to have a pain somewhere!

SCENAR FAMILY OF
DEVICES

Those of you who have read my paradigm-busting book *Virtual Medicine* (later re-published as *Medicine Beyond*) will know that I introduced the Russian SCENAR device to the world under the banner head **Star Trek Medicine Is Here!** (SCENAR is an acronym for self-controlled energo-neuro-adaptive-regulation).

Actually, it's a whole family of machines and I predicted they would completely change the face of medicine in the next 20 years. They are fast, portable, not expensive, and effective against almost any condition, especially pain, sports injuries, strokes, angina, acute infections, back pains, and irritable bowel disease, as well as pre-menstrual tension and post-surgical complications. The SCENAR even been used successfully as a portable emergency defibrillator!

Once again I have been proved right and one of the main importers to the USA tells me that now something like four out of five National Football League teams have a SCENAR device and someone trained to use it on their players. It's highly effective at resolving pain and injuries and gets the player back on the field days sooner, or even weeks sooner, than traditional first aid and rehabilitation. That's important because an injured player costs the club a fortune for every day he is incapacitated.

The device weighs around 300 gm, resembles a TV remote control, and is powered by an ordinary 9v. battery. It is placed on the skin of the chest, head, abdomen, or any diseased part, where it collects electro-magnetic signals. These are then modulated according to the on-board software program and played back to the tissues.

Charts have been developed to tell the practitioner where to place the device for its best effect.

Essentially, SCENAR is using the patient's own endogenous signals on a cybernetic feedback basis, scanning and re-transmitting many times a second. As described to me, the device "evolves" a new signal pattern for the disordered tissues, the machine literally entering into an information dialogue with the body. New frequencies and energy patterns are established, which in turn become fresh input signals, to be further modified, and so on.

This output-equals-new-input is much the way that fractals are generated and thus, biologically speaking, we seem to be on good ground here.

On the premise that disease signals are generally fixed and unnatural, anything that breaks up the existing order has the capability of disease-busting. It's certainly great for relieving pain and in the USA has been FDA-approved for that purpose.

It is emphatically not a TENS device (section 19).

History

The background to these devices is fascinating in itself and will help to give you an understanding of their capabilities.

The origin of the machine is surrounded in secrecy from the Russian military. But it clearly springs from research into the electromagnetic field effects of the body's biological energy. Eventually, a team of scientists and doctors was assembled to study possible medical applications of the technology. Researchers subsequently used it to study an Eastern therapy known as zonal contact massage.

Equipment was developed to monitor bioelectromagnetic effects taking place in the skin and use these to modulate changes in pressure of the massage. The establishment of a biofeedback mechanism led to the creation of a device whose output would depend on skin energetic response.

Through biofeedback, an interaction is formed between the tissues and the instrument; each new signal evolves as a new output. No two consecutive signals from the device are the same. This allows the treatment to be truly dynamic, adjusting for changes in the body through time and in different physiological states.

The aim with the SCENAR is to stimulate the body's own endogenous energies to effect the cure, creating a cascade of endogenous neuropeptides. This allows the body its own choice of healing ingredients; a sort of on-board pharmacy.

The Space Race

This family of healing devices was given a tremendous boost when the Soviet Union decided to send cosmonauts into orbit for prolonged periods. It was clear that they needed to have a means of treating any illnesses that could befall men who could not be rescued, except with great difficulty. Unlike the American shuttle system, there was no convenient way to bring back an ailing cosmonaut back to Earth, should the need have arisen. The possibility of incapacitating disease was a major worry.

The pharmaceutical approach was not tenable, bearing in mind the rigorous weight and space limitations in a spacecraft, and given the fact that drug-oriented medicine is based on the principle of one substance for each (potential) condition. Even a very modest therapeutic range would be weighty.

One other important consideration was that, in an environment where recycling of water is such an essential feature, any drug entering the water circulation system would remain, passing through the cosmonaut many times.

This was at a time when the Russian space program was being watched by the rest of the world and maintaining national prestige was of paramount concern to the Soviet government. It was essential to come up with something radically new. It had to be light, easy to use and, of course, really effective.

Bioenergetic technology was the only extant medical paradigm capable of delivering these stringent requirements. The SCENAR came to the fore.

Ironically, no SCENAR device has been used in space to date. There were delays caused by the authorities insisting on a waterproofing process. Before this matter was resolved, funds were suddenly stopped at the time of perestroika; the so-called "space race" was called off and the team disbanded. The USA began working on combined space projects with the Russians and they introduced the capability of evacuating sick cosmonauts on the shuttle, which meant there was no further need of on-board therapy.

Subsequent Commercialization

However, that wasn't the end of the story. Four of the original development team felt they had designed a very worthwhile system, capable of changing the face of medicine, and decided to take it onto the open market. Today, thousands of doctors in Russia are using it as their principal treatment modality and it is now available to select and trained practitioners in the West.

The promise of a small hand-held device that is capable of curing most illness, such as was portrayed in the cult 1970s TV series "Star Trek," has become a reality.

The end of the communist era led to a cessation of funding, but some of the members of the team decided to continue and formed the OKB Ritm company in 1983. Names you repeatedly come across are A.N. Revenko, Y. Grinberg, and Y. Gorfinkel, as well as lead pioneer Alexander Karasev.

They managed to get approval in 1986 from the Russian Ministry of Health for the device to be used in health clinics.

The OKB Ritm company still produces several models using names such as SCENAR 97, SCENAR NT, SCENAR 2003, Autoscenar and Kosmed. (http://www.scenar.com.ru/index_eng.html) They have a branch office in the Netherlands. (http://www.ritmedic.com/home.html)

Karasev decided to go his own way in 1990 and set up the LET Medical company, which produces a range of models under the Cosmodic brand. http://www.scenar.ru/en/)

The exception seems to be the Denas company, which decided to go down the multi-level marketing route with large numbers of resellers and reasonable prices. They have four current models, including a Euro Denas one with CE certification and an English version of their printed 240-page Denas Therapy Manual and its accompanying two-hour video, although the English translation could be much improved. Their latest model, the Diadens-DT, even includes two electro-acupuncture modes.

You can download a good 172-page English manual from the Transformation Technologies website (http://www.braintuner.com/skenar. htm). It is not stated where this manual came from, but the preface is signed Sergey Solomko; he is the owner of the Invet company.

I also discovered that there is a wealth of SCENAR-related information on the Internet but, unsurprisingly, mostly in Russian. However, I have had great success using the free online translation engine WorldLingo. (http://www.worldlingo.com/en/products_services/worldlingo_translator.html)

Google also do their own translator page. Incidentally, my name will come up with 46 million returns, if you Google for "star trek medicine scott-mumby" (*as of May 23, 2014*).

So How Does It Work?

As I said, the model is that of stimulating the on-board pharmacy of our brain. That includes the release of endorphins, our natural morphine-like compounds. It performs better with a skilled operator, of course. But it's remarkably good for self-healing. Applications include dental pain, headache, sore throat, bruises, arthritis, injuries, and fractures.

In fact, it is quite exceptional for pain relief. I have seen a SCENAR dispel severe biliary colic, toothache, and the pain of a fracture through the ankle in a matter of minutes (biliary colic—gallstones—is one of medicine's two worst pains; the other is a kidney stone).

The SCENAR also adapts very well with acupuncture (section 6) and the auriculo-acupuncture method of Nogier (section 7).

In the right hands, a SCENAR can also be skillfully combined with knowledge of myofascial trigger points. These are said to be the origin of a great deal of soft-tissue pain. The trigger point may not be where the pain is felt (referred pain) so it took a little time for this phenomenon to come to light (section 11).

Here are some examples of what can be achieved:

Casebook

1. Male, 69 years old

This man, who was a gardener by profession, had chronic suppurating osteomyelitis of the foot that could not be controlled. He was scheduled for an amputation of the lower leg in four days time, largely due to intractable pain that had lasted over a year. Someone decided to try a SCENAR device on him. It was run over the affected limb for about 30 minutes.

Next day, the pain had vanished for the first time in eight months. Later that day, another 30-minute treatment was given. By next morning the recovery was so dramatic that the amputation was called off. A third treatment was given and seven days after the first SCENAR this man was back at work, digging in the garden. His leg has completely recovered.

2. Female, age 68 years

This lady had attended for successful treatment of her asthma. She commented on painful arthritic knees. I decided to try the SCENAR. In order to gauge the effectiveness of the treatment, I suggested that we concentrate on the left knee only and she could compare any improvements with the status of the right knee.

Next morning she rang and was delighted that the pain had vanished from BOTH knees. One week later, as of the time she returned to the UK, she had no further pain.

Pets

It's great for animals, too. Roger Meacock, a UK veterinary, uses one routinely in his practice and has found it very helpful for keeping valuable racehorses in condition when they have suffered sprains or injuries.

My friend Lorraine (Lorry) Ann Vanbergen from Vancouver Island has a nice story to tell about her pet dog Alexi, a 10-month old Pomeranian, who had as broken leg with three separate fractures. The vet's options were not good: basically, an amputation or a metal plate. She decided to use the SCENAR instead; Lorry is one of the main international teachers of SCENAR therapy.

The limb was put in a cast and Lorry worked on the healthy limb on the other side. Suffice it to say that Alexi made a rapid recovery, which quite amazed the veterinary.

The key points are:
- The rapid healing
- The comfort and freedom from any real pain

Clinical Aspects

The SCENAR device is very safe because the impulse times are very short. No pain is felt but the patient is usually aware of a tingling sensation while it works. The practitioner seeks what the Russians term asymmetry, meaning something different about the tissue characteristics in the vicinity. There are five main criteria:

- discoloration (reddening or pallor)
- sensation (numbness or hyper-aesthesia)
- stickiness, in which the machine drags with a magnet-like quality as it is drawn over certain tracts of the skin
- sound changes (the machine begins to chatter electronically as it hits certain zones)
- change in numerical output display

Even though it may not coincide with the obvious area of pain or pathology, the important point is to treat the asymmetry. This is similar to the use of trigger points or "interference fields" in neural therapy; we treat what the body is offering, not necessarily the site of the pain.

For reasons we do not fully understand, when the asymmetry is eliminated, recovery will rapidly follow.

There are remarkably few contra-indications, notably heart pacemakers and, after 20 years, a complete absence of negative side effects. SCENAR technology can be used as a valuable addition to other therapies or can be a stand-alone treatment.

A brilliant device indeed!

The Avazzia

We now have another family of SCENAR-type devices, the Avazzia, made in Texas, USA (not to be confused with Jerry Tennant's copycat devices, also from Texas). These are of good build quality and come accompanied with intelligible instructions, not pidgin English!

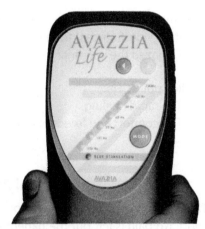

Everything said above about the SCENAR can apply equally well to the Avazzia, including the fact that they are FDA-approved. Their onboard software is known by the acronym BEST (biofeedback electro-stimulation technology). This non-pharmaceutical, non-invasive technology is designed to stimulate the body's natural release of nitric oxide, endorphins and neuropeptides into the blood stream.

Nitric oxide causes vascular dilation and thereby increases blood circulation. This is critical to wound healing, reduction of edema, elimination of irritant metabolites, and thus pain relief.

As a result, the Avazzia family are able to provide quick relief of chronic and acute pains. Moreover, pain relief is long-lasting: up to 12 hours, and frequently longer, which is good news for sufferers.

Nitric oxide, by the way, is also great for cerebral blood flow and erectile function (Viagra works only by blocking the breakdown of nitric oxide).

One extra valuable detail: BEST technology is designed to continually modify waveforms to prevent the body becoming habituated to the signals (or becoming accommodated, as we say). This phenomenon of the body getting used to something bedevils a lot of therapeutic modalities. As a result, a treatment which works well at first may eventually cease to provide much benefit.

The Avazzia people claim to have conquered this impediment.

So, these devices are not exactly cheap but they are reasonably priced. It's an investment in your family's health for a whole lifetime. Every home should have one, is my motto! The perfect answer to pain, easy, FAST and effective.

Lorraine and her husband, John Hache, Doctor of Natural Medicine and a Naturopathic Physician, can be found at: www.PacificHealthOptions. com and www.AvazziaLife.com I have no hesitation in recommending them. They offer devices and provide top quality training.

LIGHT THERAPY FOR PAIN

For centuries scientists have devoted untiring effort to discover a means for the relief or cure of human ills and restoration of the normal functions. Yet in neglected light and color there is a potency far beyond that of drugs and serums.

—Kate W. Baldwin,
M.D., EA.C.S., Fellow, American Medical Association.

Now we come to another surprise healing modality that you can try for almost any kind of pain: the use of light!

Among the earliest writers to advocate light therapy were Herodotus, Galen, and the great Arabian physician Avicenna. The ancient Egyptians used a type of color therapy. But the Greeks went further in both the theory and practice of light medicine, using the sun's rays to treat disease in the famous healing temples of Heliopolis (Sun City).

In our own century, Nobel laureate Albert Szent-Gyorgi (who discovered vitamin C) acknowledges the profound influence of light on our health and states and that all the energy we take into our bodies is derived directly or indirectly from the sun. Ultimately, all life energy derives from the sun. It is correct to speak of light as a nutrient.

But Szent-Gyorgi took it much further than this. His research concluded that many of the body's enzymes and hormones are functionally sensitive to light. Color changes can significantly affect the power and effectiveness of these enzymes and hormones. His findings were subsequently verified by researchers Martinek and Berezin in 1979, who found that some colors can increase the activity of enzymes by up to 500 per cent and markedly affect the transport of chemicals across cell membranes. It has even been found that the absence of certain wavelengths in light results in the body being unable to absorb fully all dietary nutrients.

Throw Away That Sunscreen!

Rays from our Sun are among the most healing properties of Nature. Sunshine has been shown to heal wounds and kill microbes. It's known as the "Florence Nightingale effect."

Yet sunshine has a bad rap these days. Ignorant, stupid and dangerous "science" prompts the advice to stay out of the sun. Or, if you must go to the beach, slather yourself in carcinogenic sunblock creams.

The truth is that *real* science shows that sunshine protects from cancer, it does not cause it. In 1999, I specifically quoted an Australian study (they should know), published in the prestigious medical journal *Lancet*, showing that the incidence of malignant melanoma was far higher in office workers than in those who were regularly exposed to sunlight due to lifestyle or occupation. In other words, living and working in the sun was beneficial. [Beral V, et al. Malignant melanoma and exposure to fluorescent light. *Lancet* 2 (1982): 290-292.]

It doesn't stop there. The advice to stay out of the sun or block sunlight with sunscreen is the worst advice you can get for your prostate. A study also published in the Lancet (2001), showed that the group that got the least exposure to the ultraviolet rays of the sun were *three times more likely* to develop prostate cancer than those in the group that got the most sun exposure.

The people who had the highest sunlight exposure reduced their risk of developing prostate cancer by 66 percent. [Luscombe C, et. al. Exposure to ultraviolet radiation: association with susceptibility and age at presentation with prostate cancer. *The Lancet;* 2001; 358; 9282; 641-642.]

Another study in a different journal (*Anticancer Research*) showed that sunlight exposure alone — about 20 minutes a day for fair-skinned folks and two to four times that much for those with dark skin — can reduce the risk of prostate cancer and 15 other types of cancer in both men and women. [Grant W, et. al. The association of solar ultraviolet B (UVB) with reducing risk of cancer: multifactorial ecologic analysis of geographic variation in age-adjusted cancer mortality rates. *Anticancer Research*. 2006; 26:2687-2700.]

Sunlight Is Our Healing Friend

I'm saying this to point out that sunlight has beneficial and protective properties. Ignorance (and no doubt the influence of the sunscreen market dollars) has demonized it as dangerous.

Little wonder, then, that lack of light can have severely destructive health consequences and that, conversely, the right kind of light can prove enormously healing. Just sitting in the warm relaxing sun can ease your pain; it's a common experience.

It is important not to forget that light is just another electromagnetic energy form. The fact that we can see it gives us a deep psychological relationship to light, but it is really no different in quality from radio waves or x-rays. Because of this, we can gain a glimpse of what detailed information may be contained in light energy form; just think of the information carried to radios and TVs.

There are several useful pain treatments which employ light including, of course, lasers (section 14). In this section we will look at three specific adaptations of light energy, including the use of color, gemstones, and special electronic machines that can deliver other EM frequencies.

Let's start with the simplest of these…

Color Therapy (Chromotherapy)

White full-spectrum light is now being used in the treatment of cancers, SAD (seasonal affective disorder), anorexia, bulimia, insomnia, jet lag, shift-working, and alcohol and drug dependency.

Different colored light has a profound effect on how we feel and how a space feels (room lighting) and has important symbolic meaning, such as in art.

Experimental research lends support to these observations. Viewing red light has been found to increase subjects' strength by 13.5 percent and to elicit 5.8 percent more electrical activity in the arm muscles. For this reason it is now used to improve the performance of athletes. Whereas red light appears to help athletes who need short, quick bursts of energy, blue light assists in performances requiring a more steady energy output.

By comparison, pink has been found to have a tranquilizing and calming effect within minutes of exposure. It suppresses hostile, aggressive, and anxious behavior — interesting, given its traditional association with women in Western culture. Pink holding cells are now widely used to reduce violent and aggressive behavior among prisoners, and some sources have reported a reduction of muscle strength in inmates within 2.7 seconds. It appears that, when in pink surroundings, people cannot be aggressive even if they want to, because the color saps their energy.

A special application of light energies we call chromotherapy or color therapy. Briefly, different colors have different energetic qualities and each is healing in its own way.

In 1990, scientists reported to the annual conference of the American Association for the Advancement of Science on the successful use of blue light in the treatment of a wide variety of psychological problems, including addictions, eating disorders, impotence, and depression.

Blue light has also been shown effective in the treatment of arthritis pain. In studies by S. F. McDonald, most of those exposed to blue light for variable periods up to 15 minutes experienced a significant degree of pain relief. It was concluded that the pain reduction was directly related both to the blue light and the length of exposure to it.

In fact, blue light can heal injured tissue and prevent scar tissue, in the treatment of cancers and nonmalignant tumors, as well as skin and lung conditions.

American Civil War General Augustus Pleasonton (1801-1894) conducted his own experiments and in 1876 published his book *The Influence of the Blue Ray of the Sunlight and of the Blue Color of the Sky* about how the color blue can improve the growth of crops and livestock and can help heal diseases in humans.

Blue light seems to be the big one, but other colors which have a known effect on pain include dark yellow and violet/deep purple. Avicenna (980-1037), no less, wrote that yellow light cools and soothes inflammation and reduces muscular pain.

Here's what you can do:

Chromotherapy is administered with the use of special color filters. The benchmark has always been Dinshah Ghadiali filters, using his original five matched colored glass plates to produce 12 Spectro-Chrome colors, as described in the paradigm book, *Let There Be Light*.

However, color gels seem to be virtually as good. You can buy inexpensive kits of 4 x 4 or 6 x 6 Eleven Roscolene Color Filters of a very specific and closely matched hue (color frequency), which have been found to achieve the same therapeutic results obtained by the Ghadiali set.

Ken Adachi has assembled the filters you need and is offering them as a set on this page: http://educate-yourself.org/products/index.shtml; scroll down to the heading: Spectro-Chrome Light Therapy.

You might also like to get a copy of the book by William Campbell Douglas MD, *Color Me Healthy with 6.5' x 6.5' Roscolene Color Filters*, which can be found on Amazon

Caution

Just remember blue isn't always good; at the wrong time of day it has adverse effects by disjointing our circadian rhythms.

Here's what Nature does:

- In the mornings, we awake to yellow light (that delicious golden glow of sunrise!)
- At mid-day, when we are at our most active, blue light is dominant.
- In the evening, mellowed reddish colors calm and prepare us for sleep.

Red light encourages the release of melatonin, our "sleep hormone" (blue light suppresses this vital, healthy rest hormone).

The answer is to have a variety of colored lamps, bulbs and shades. Use photographic gels, if you can't do it any other way.

- Put on yellow light in the morning.
- Switch to blue during the working day
- Go orange in the late afternoon and warm red for the evenings.

The ultimate smart lighting system is coming: you walk into your house, the sensor system detects who you are and what you need, and adjusts the lights accordingly. Your alarm clock could turn on your bedroom light in yellow wake-up mode in the morning.

Aurvedic Gem Elixir Therapy

In a parallel tradition, which actually predates ours, ayurvedic medicine also has a light healing system.

It's based on gemstones. Quite simply, "soaking" water in gemstones, using light as the "propellant," has immense and proven health benefits. OK, that didn't sound very scientific, so what do I mean really?

The practice is to put certain gems into water and place the bottle in direct sunlight for a few days, for the gem "essence" to imprint in the water. Of course, gems are solids and don't have an essence or odor. But they do have a characteristic vibrational frequency, which can be imparted to the water. This is the "elixir."

You could use a sapphire ring of your own and just place it in water (maybe with a few drops of vodka or brandy, like a homeopathic remedy) and stand it on the kitchen windowsill for a week.

There's a whole system on which this is based and certain discoveries, which are replicatable. For example, sapphire is cooling and soothing, so is emerald; both are analgesic. Diamond is very energizing; so is ruby. Carnelian has antiseptic properties and citrine is warm, enlivening and cleansing.

Ayurvedic gem therapy views disease and disharmony as basically color starvation; the "excited" liquid of the elixir rectifies the energy deficit. You know, the huge bejewelled rings that were worn by Indian princes, nabobs, and potentates were not always merely for the display of wealth and self-aggrandizement! Some rings were intended for therapeutic purposes. Such a ring had no back, so that sunlight could shine straight through the precious stone and so irradiate the skin and tissues beneath with beneficial rays

Powders

The other major traditional route of administration was using ground-up gem powders. I wrote in my 1999 book *Virtual Medicine* that this is not to be recommended (apart from the cost). These substances can be very powerful emanators and modulators of quantum electromagnetic energy, as we shall see below, and should be regarded seriously as such. Introducing solid substances which perhaps may never be removed or excreted fully from the body, but can go on causing harm if they are the wrong choice, may prove disastrous.

Even when we understand these things much better than we do now, it still lacks sensible rationale, as these gem powders may pre-empt any possibility of changing modalities as the body's state or disease process alters.

Readers who wish to experiment with gem elixirs should make them up as described above and not take the solid form – even if cost is no object!

Not Color Therapy

Unfortunately, this fascinating yet cogent discipline has too long languished and is still little known outside its country of origin. Modern light therapists and researchers such as Jacob Liberman and John Ott seem to ignore it. But with the advancement of science and the ability to translate older methods from a stultifying background into a modern framework and quantifiable results, we may say "gem therapy" has indeed come of age and will grow steadily in applications in the West.

Despite superficial similarities, gem therapy is not crystal therapy. Quartz, amethyst, tourmaline, moonstone, and many other commonly used therapeutic crystals the reader may have heard about seem to have little or no value in this "light-stressing" context.

Nor is it exactly color therapy. Tests show that the color of the light is irrelevant. In other words, it is the gem that dictates the resulting effect and not its color, as perceived by the patient. This is odd, since the Indian tradition regards the need for gems and their effectiveness as being evidence of color starvation.

The Electronic Approach

So far, so good. But is there a better way?

In this techno-advanced, quantum-aware world, you might wonder if there is something more powerful and, perhaps, easier to use. There is.

Probably the most advanced instrument of this type today is the Stellar Delux, developed by electronics engineer Jon Whale. The Stellar Delux supercedes his earlier instruments the Caduceus Lux, Lux III & IV which were developed in the 1990's.

The essence of Whale's approach is that when gem stones are electronically excited their crystalline structure vibrates at the atomic level and emit energy. By containing a quantity of gem stones inside an electronic frequency controlled transducer lamp, the gem energy produced can be transmitted and directed in such a way to accurately target diseased or injured parts of the body.

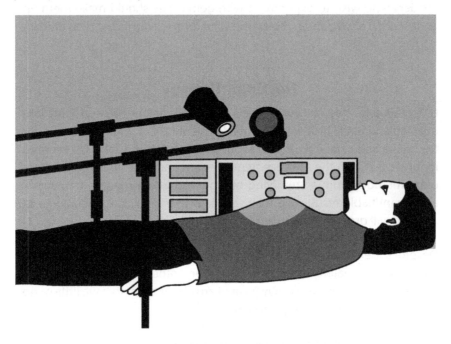

The gem energy is directly transmitted by 'dielectric resonance' to diseased or injured tissue bones, organs or glands. In addition, the colored filtered light photons passing through the gem stone chamber within the transducer becomes 'modulated' with the characteristics of the gems, as with the gem elixir therapy just described. The changes to the light are probably at the quantum level and we are unable to measure them scientifically yet. But the body tissues can detect the changes and react differently to each type of light in a most remarkable and consistent fashion.

A everyday example of 'dielectric resonance transmission' is the 'Piezo-electricity' that is generated within a quartz crystal frequency oscillator an essential component in TV's computers, watches, clocks, radio transmitters, etc..

The important point to grasp is that all dielectric electromagnetic waves including light travels very far into the tissues. The experience of shining a torch through your hand on a dark night will tell you this; even a small wattage of a 3-volt battery torch will make the back of the hand glow red as the blood vessels and deep tissue are illuminated. The Stellar Delux electronic gem therapy lamps use high-intensity bulbs. The powerful beam is filtered and focused through lenses and consequently has far more penetration. Light will pass into the chest, abdomen, and major bones and even penetrate the skull.

What you feel when you put your hand into the beam is a distinct and palpable pressure from the radiation. It is an astonishing thing to experience. Whale has designed lamps that house the gems in the path of the light and concentrate it in a useful beam. The whole apparatus is simple to use and produces results that are little short of sensational. Recoveries range from breast lumps to arthritis, eczema to colitis.

BUT—and here's the beauty of the device—it isn't merely the "gem quality" of the light that creates the therapeutic effect. Whale's innovative idea was to develop a machine which allowed programming of the incident light with brain wave frequencies (delta, theta, etc).

So the light shone through the gem chamber could then be modulated by electronically exciting gem stones with theta frequency (4 – 8 Hertz), which is calming, relaxing and dreamy. In fact delta frequency (1 - 3 Hertz) is the brainwave equivalent to sleep or unconsciousness, in other words, total anesthesia!

I have owned and used this equipment myself (the Lux IV and Stellar Delux are similar but the latter even more powerful) so I can speak from direct experience. I have seen it work amazing changes in a matter of minutes. It is especially good for acute injuries. The fiery heat of swelling, vasodilation and pain calms rapidly, under the soothing influence of emerald and dark blue sapphire. This has been confirmed, using infrared thermography imaging. In addition, we can modulate the light signal to the slow analgesic frequency of sleep (1.5 Hertz) being employed for a large percentage presented disease or injury.

Gem Properties

A fuller list of commonly-used gems and their properties is given, to complete this section:

Gem	Color	Properties
Carnelian	Orange	Cooling, moist and harmonizing, anti-allergic
Chrysoberyl	Infra-red	Hot, penetrating, cleansing, deep heating
Citrine	Yellow	Warm, enlivening, cleansing

Diamond	Indigo	Stimulating, invigorating, clarifying, anti-depressant
Emerald	Green	Cold, unifying and solidifying, analgesic
Ruby	Red	Heating, drying, energizing, expanding
Sapphire	Violet	Tranquillizing, soothing, analgesic, antispasmodic
Topaz	Blue	Cool, soft, satisfying, antiseptic

Casebook: Female, 45 Years

A woman therapist had torn a muscle in an amateur stage production. The noise of the muscle rupture was so loud it was heard in the second row. She was promptly incapacitated and in great pain.

She came to see me a few days later, limping badly, all other attempts at therapy having failed. I gave her first a routine 20 minutes of calming and relaxation, with emerald-sapphire stones at 3.3 Hz. This very aware patient was able to tell me that her pelvis underwent a shift back into the normal energetic position during this stage of treatment.

I followed through with about 30 minutes to the injured calf. All pain had now vanished from the affected leg, but a new pain had appeared in the opposite knee. This was probably due to the stress of limping and bearing all her weight on that side, but the pain had, of necessity, been suppressed. Now it emerged (common response to successful therapy of all kinds).

A further 15 minutes on the uninjured side removed that discomfort too, and the patient walked to her car with no discernible limp. Next day she phoned to say there was only mild discomfort, she was back at work and she was content with just one treatment.

You can find out more about this amazing device at Whale Medical: http://www.whalemedical.com/

LASERS

We all know one of the buzzwords for advanced technology is the laser. It is coherent light, produced synthetically; it does not exist in nature, except as ultra-weak luminescence. I have indicated that this may be the defining nature of living tissue.

Low-level laser therapy (LLLT) uses low-power lasers (or even light-emitting diodes) to alter biological function. Other names for this therapy include low-power laser, soft laser and cold laser. High-power lasers, by contrast, will burn and kill tissue, while low-power lasers may stimulate cells to function.

The ability of LLLT to relieve pain is beyond dispute. This can extend to:
- Plantar fasciitis
- Neuropathies
- Arthritis (osteo- and rheumatoid)
- Acute and chronic neck pain
- Sports injuries
- Tendon & ligament injuries
- Back & joint pain
- Muscle sprains & strains
- Tendonitis
- Post-surgical swelling
- Disc compression
- Sore muscles

Other clinical benefits include:
- Anti-inflammatory effect
- Accelerated tissue repair and cell growth
- Improved blood flow
- Increases metabolic activity
- Stimulation of trigger points and acupuncture points
- Reduced fibrous tissue formation
- Improved nerve function
- Faster wound healing

In other words, we have here a pretty useful addition to the weaponry against pain. Lasers are effective at treating a wide variety of conditions, including soft-tissue injuries, acute injuries, or nerve damage. They key points are ease of use, safety, and efficacy.

It is unclear exactly how LLLT works. It may reduce pain related to inflammation by lowering levels of inflammatory cytokines, oxidative stress, edema, and bleeding.

Another postulated mechanism may be related to stimulation of mitochondria to increase the production of adenosine triphosphate, resulting in an increase in reactive oxygen species, which influences redox signaling, affecting intracellular homeostasis or the proliferation of cells. If that sounds too technical for you, don't worry about it. Medically-trained practitioners will grasp it.

Dosage

The effect of a laser device seems to be related to two main functions: power (in milliwatts) and wavelength (penetration).

A higher-powered laser is a brighter light, and it can produce more energy per unit of time. Most useful devices are in the range of 500 milliwatts. Less than that would be equivalent to a laser pointer, rather than a therapeutic device.

It seems that below a certain power level, LLLT has no effect whatever. In other words, there is a minimum threshold.

Wavelength is critical and needs to be in the red band: range 600-1000 nm (red to near infrared), but some research has been done and products outside of this range are available. Notably, this includes the powerful wavelength of 635 nm.

A wavelength of 635 nm is significant in that it has well-known and documented anti-inflammatory effects by inhibiting cyclooxygenase (COX) and prostaglandin PGE2, much like powerful COXs inhibitor (see page 25). However 635 nm light also protects against oxidative stress damage; NSAIDs do not.

Many devices work nearer to 800 nm, which penetrates several centimeters into the body and will reach most tissue injuries.

Also influencing the value-outcome is the phenomenon of pulses (peak power and repetition rates), which is still poorly understood in the clinical setting

Doses are usually measured in joules per sq. centimeter. A range between 0.3 and 19 joules per sq. cm. appear to be most appropriate.

Times are on the order of 20 minutes. You will not likely get full relief or resolution from pain symptoms after just one treatment. It takes a series of sessions, usually 8 to 30, depending on the severity and duration of the condition.

Laser Classes

Lasers are classified according to their power output:
- Class 3a—maximum of 5 milliwatts of power (standard laser pointer)
- Class 3b—maximum of 500 milliwatts
- Class 4—anything over 500 milliwatts

Some practitioners make the mistake of using a low-power Class 3 laser, which basically amounts to a standard laser pointer.

Most class 3a lasers only use a red wavelength – 635 nanometers in the visible red. Red light penetrates poorly, compared to blue. Consequently, red laser light only penetrates about one to two millimeters (far less than 1/8 inch) into the human body. This is useful for treating superficial wounds, cuts, abrasions, and perhaps even for the treatment of vitiligo.

For deeper penetration, such as deep-seated pain reduction, around 800 nanometers (infrared) is needed and is able to go several centimeters into the body and reach most tissue injuries. That needs more power and a Class 4 infrared laser is the benchmark treatment to reduce pain, reduce inflammation, and enhance tissue healing—both in hard and soft tissues, including muscles, ligaments, or even bones.

In addition, correct treatment stimulates the cytochrome oxidase enzyme in the mitochondria of the cells. This is really one of the key discoveries in the whole science of laser therapy. Specifically, injured cells are targeted because damaged cells are more readily accepting of photons of light, whereas healthy cells don't need this extra energy.

Intra-Nasal Laser Light

A great modern idea for applying laser light, without the need for any office visit, is via the intranasal route. The healing light is literally shone up the nostril. It works well, because the nasal passages are especially richly supplied with blood vessels and have a high blood flow (turnover rate).

Actually, red light LEDs work almost as well in the 635 nm range. But for faster, surer results, low level lasers work better and are only slightly more costly.

VieLight, one of the leaders in this field, have a range of products, including a 635 nm. LED model, a 655 nm low level laser model. They also provide accessories that allow light to be shone directly onto injured or painful tissues, and spare nasal applicators, so others don't have to share what's been up your nose!.

Learn more about this highly effective pain-healing modality here: www.alternative-doctor.com/pain

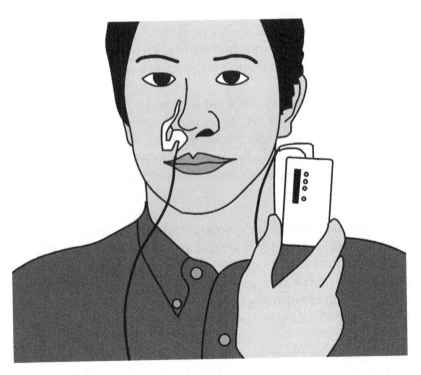

Cost

These devices are majorly inexpensive, considering their capabilities. Treatments are short, so an office visit will not be prohibitive.

Laser therapy can be effectively combined with a number of other treatment modalities, including various soft tissue mobilization techniques. The laser treatment is best done first.

If you make a purchase, do make sure there is good instruction with it. You will not likely succeed without at least a short participatory course.

Paradox Medicine

Now we turn to something almost unique, based on the very special capability of lasers to hold and transmit biological information.

Performance scientist Ken West discovered a way to use lasers to pump healing homeopathic information into the body via acupuncture points. Remedies that work well by mouth will work even faster by this route, which is a valuable advance where immediate treatment of sports injuries is of essence. If this sounds a little bizarre, I may tell you that Ken has been retained by a number of sports clubs, who don't like to waste money! They would only consider a remedy approach if it actually delivered cost-effective results.

It started with the work of Prof. Yoshito Mukaino, of Fukuoka University, showing a 20% increase in ball speed of athletes, as a result of balancing acupuncture meridians (acupuncture, see section 6). Mukaino's work has now become widely accepted and many athletes around the world use his "Meridian Test."

Realizing that acupuncture points are a natural "window" to the body tissues, Ken worked with Dr. Dane Oosthuizen to develop a therapy system called "Paradox Medicine," using acupuncture combined with a knowledge of homeopathy. In this case, Ken knows well the Reckeweg repertoire of formulas from HEEL (Baden-Baden, see section 8).

Experimenting with a hand-held laser gun, Ken simply shines light through the remedy onto the skin, at suitable sites (this is remedies in small glass phials). Remarkably, the "information" imprint of the remedy is transferred to the tissues, with very beneficial healing results.

Remember, this is about tissue repair and healing, not analgesia as such. However, I have observed rapid pain reduction and it is a more intelligent way to reduce tissue inflammation and discomfort, than merely masking it with blunderbuss painkillers.

For reasons that are not quite clear, this seems to work better if Japanese acupuncture (Jin Shan) points are used. These are fewer in number than the Chinese points and, although there is some overlap, are rather different. Ken describes the Japanese points as "deeper" and reverts to Chinese points if the patient is young, old, or weak.

Ken's work is further interesting to me in that he has boiled the entire HEEL repertory of remedies down to about a dozen items. By examining diligently each of the HEEL compounded remedies, he found many contained the same substances, grouped in different ways. By using a much narrower range of products, he was able to administer to his patients almost the complete repertory.

Ken West's "Library"

Ken divides his travel kit into three groups of master remedies and three related remedies for each, making a list of 12 in all. For those of you who are practitioners and may wish to explore this concept, I list them here, as follows:

Group Remedy	Related Remedies
Galium-HEEL® group	Thyroidea compositum
	Cerebrum compositum
	Mucosa Compositum
Traumeel® group	Echinacea compositum
	Engystol compositum
	Lymphomyosot
Coenzyme compositum® group	Ubichinon compositum
	Hepar compositum
	Zeel

All HEEL product names are subject to trademark. See more about Traumeel on page 53.

In discussion with Ken, I told him I would add one other super-defense and tissue-strengthening remedy and Ken agreed: Discus compositum®. It's especially recommended for joint disorders, including chronic arthritis, neuralgic and rheumatic disorders, exhaustion, and debility. This sounds like a plug for HEEL, I know, but they are good.

Ken offered a useful tip for those practitioners who feel they may be encountering tissue stress, as a result of heavy detoxing: the use of homeopathically potentized vitamin B3 (niacin; don't use niacinamide). This makes sense to me, since niacin is a key precursor to NADH detox path- ways; a strong reducing agent.

HEEL products can be obtained from:

Biologische Heilmittel Heel GmbH
Dr. Reckeweg-Straße 2-4
76532 Baden-Baden
Telephone: +49 07221
E-Mail: info@heel.de

Or through national distributors, such as **Biopathica UK** (who also supply Russia):
PO Box 217, Ashford, Kent, TN23 6ZU
Phone: +44 (0)1233 636678
Email: products@biopathica.co.uk

Some, but not all, can be obtained from:
HEEL USA in Albuquerque, New Mexico.
Heel, Inc.
10421 Research Road SE
Albuquerque, NM 87123-3423
1-800-920-9203 or 505-293-3843
Email Inquiries:
info@heelusa.com

HYPNOTHERAPY

People don't need hypnotizing, they are already hypnotized. They need un-hypnotizing, says hypnotist Jack True. People need waking up and that was the message of Russian mystic genius George Gurdjieff. People are asleep.

Notwithstanding, we all know—or think we know—the power of hypnotism to change a person's point of view.

There's a common misconception that this can be done in a sneaky fashion, without the person being aware of it or giving permission. This is simply not true. The patient has to cooperate. Forget the Svengali angle.

Hypnosis in the treatment of chronic pain generally, but not always, involves a hypnotic induction with suggestions for relaxation and comfort. Posthypnotic suggestions may be given for reduced pain that can continue beyond the session so that the patient can quickly and easily create a state of comfort using a cue (i.e., taking a deep breath and exhaling as eye lids close).

The focus of hypnosis in the treatment of chronic pain also often involves teaching the patient self-hypnosis or providing tape recordings of hypnosis sessions that can be used to reduce pain on a daily basis outside the sessions. Some patients experience an immediate reduction in pain severity following hypnosis treatment, whereas others can obtain reduction in pain with repeated practice of self-hypnosis or hypnosis sessions.

Research shows that hypnosis works as part of a treatment program for a number of psychological and medical conditions, with pain relief being one of the most researched areas, as shown in a 2000 study by psychologists Steven Lynn, PhD; Irving Kirsch, PhD; Arreed Barabasz, PhD; Etzel Cardeña, PhD; and David Patterson, PhD.

Hypnosis has been applied to a variety of chronic-pain conditions, including those from cancer, low-back problems, arthritis, sickle cell disease, temporomandibular joint conditions, fibromyalgia, physical disability and various other pains of mixed origins. [*Int J Clin Exp Hypn.* (Jul 2007); 55(3): 275–287.]

Among the benefits associated with hypnosis is the ability to alter the psychological components of the experience of pain that may then have an effect on even severe pain. This is called hypno-analgesia.

In their 2003 review of controlled clinical studies, Dr. Patterson and fellow psychologist Mark Jensen, PhD, found that hypno-analgesia is associated with significant reductions in ratings of pain, need for analgesics or sedation, nausea and vomiting, and length of stay in hospitals.

Hypnosis has also been associated with better overall outcome after medical treatment and greater physiological stability. Surgeons and other health providers have reported significantly higher degrees of satisfaction with their patients treated with hypnosis than with their other patients.

Patients who are most receptive to hypnotic suggestions in general, or highly hypnotizable, have found the greatest and most lasting relief from hypnosis techniques, but people with moderate suggestibility (the majority of people) also show improvement. Factors such as motivation and compliance with treatment may also affect responsiveness to hypnotic suggestions. As I said, the patient has to be on board, not tricked into changing their perceptions.

Drs. Patterson and Jensen's review also concluded that hypnotism for acute pain is very superior to and often better than other recognized treatments for pain. [Patterson DR, Jensen MP. Hypnosis and clinical pain. *Psychological Bulletin.* 2003; 129: 495-521.]

Another analysis of studies from 2000 concluded that 75% of clinical and experimental participants with different types of pain obtained substantial pain relief from hypnotic techniques. Thus, hypnosis is likely to be effective for most people suffering from diverse forms of pain, with the possible exception of a minority of patients who are resistant to hypnotic interventions.

[Montgomery GH, DuHamel KN, Redd WH. A meta-analysis of hypnotically induced analgesia: How effective is hypnosis? *International Journal of Clinical and Experimental Hypnosis.* 2000; 48: 138-153.]

Practical Application

Hypno-analgesia has been used successfully in a number of interventions in many clinics, hospitals, and burn care centers, and dental offices. For acute pain, it has proven effective in interventional radiology, various surgical procedures (e.g., appendectomies, tumor excisions), the treatment of burns (dressing changes and the painful removal of dead or contaminated skin tissue), childbirth labor pain, bone marrow aspiration pain, and pain related to dental work, especially so with children.

Chronic pain conditions for which hypnosis has been used successfully include, among others, headache, backache, fibromyalgia, carcinoma-related pain, temporomandibular disorder pain, and mixed chronic pain.

Moreover, hypnosis can alleviate the sensory and/or affective components of a pain experience, which may be all that is required for acute pain.

Chronic conditions, however, may require a comprehensive plan that targets various aspects besides the pain experience. The patient may need help increasing behaviors that foster well-being and functional activity (e.g., exercise, good diet) challenging faulty thinking patterns (e.g., "I cannot do anything about my pain"), restoring range of motion and appropriate body mechanics, and so on.

Cancer Pain

If you are suffering from pain due to cancer and its invasions, this is certainly one to consider.

A 1983 study, for example, found hypno-analgesia and other post-hypnotic suggestions very helpful; 54 women with chronic cancer pain from breast carcinoma were assigned to either standard care or weekly expressive-supportive group therapy for up to 12 months. The women entered in the group therapy were divided: some had hypnosis training as a part of their treatment, some did not.

The hypnosis intervention was directed toward enhancing patient competence and mastery in managing pain and stress related to cancer. Hypnotic training included suggestions to "filter out the hurt" of any sensations by imagining competing sensations in affected areas.

Patients were also given instructions for using self-hypnosis outside of the group-therapy sessions.

Both treatment groups demonstrated significantly less pain and suffering than the control sample. The authors ask us to note that hypnosis was not the main focus of the expressive-supportive group-therapy sessions, but the patients who received hypnosis in addition to group therapy reported significantly less increase in pain over time (as cancer progressed), compared to patients who did not receive the hypnosis intervention. [Spiegel D, Bloom JR. Group therapy and hypnosis reduce metastatic breast carcinoma pain. *Psychosomatic Medicine*. 1983; 45: 333–339.]

In another study published in 2004, 39 patients with advanced-stage cancer (Stage III or IV) were entered into a randomized study. Patients were randomly assigned to receive either weekly sessions of supportive attention or a hypnosis intervention.

The hypnosis intervention involved at least four weekly sessions, which included suggestions for relaxation, comfort, mental imagery for dissociation and pain control, and instruction in self-hypnosis. In addition, patients in the hypnosis intervention were provided with an audiocassette tape recording of a hypnotic induction and instructed in home practice of hypnosis.

The hypnosis intervention group demonstrated a significant overall decrease in pain for all sessions combined. Interestingly, the effectiveness of self-hypnosis practice outside the sessions was separately evaluated and came out at 6.5 on a scale of 1 - 10. [Elkins GR, Cheung A, Marcus J, Palamara L, Rajab H. Hypnosis to reduce pain in cancer survivors with advanced disease: A prospective study. *J Cancer Integrative Medicine*. 2004; 2: 167–172.]

If you want to know about clinical studies demonstrating the effects of hypnosis on various types of pain, a very good article in the *International Journal of Clinical and Experimental Hypnosis* (2007) summarized many good trials and included a good list of citations. [*Int J Clin Exp Hypn*. Jul 2007; 55(3): 275–287.]

Specific Techniques for You to Try

We now need to go forward and look at some specific techniques. For that I call upon my friend and expert hypnotherapist, Elaine Kissel. She has three powerful suggestions.

Technique number one: Imagine the pain in some tangible form. It doesn't matter what it is (although a symbolic form is most helpful); think of it as solid matter, the size you can get hold of, and put it in a box, along with its causes, of course. Be sure to feel the power you have to contain the pain, to handle it, to be in control of it. Then seal the box, feel yourself forcing the lid down, locking it tightly, and throw it away. Cast it into outer space or whatever distant location you want. Put it in a bottomless pit. Discard it with a sense of absolute finality. Feel your determination in this endeavor. Be sure to sense that you are in control of this pain, and you are getting rid of it.

A dispassionate attitude can be quite helpful here as it helps you to disengage your fears and other unhelpful emotions. For some people, this "cold-hearted" approach works better than an emotional one. Some people need to be angry with the pain, to get up enough courage to face the pain from a position of strength and to overpower the fear with the kind of anger that revs up their resolve.

However, if it is fear you are getting rid of, you need to overpower it with another kind of emotion. Certain emotions, such as anger, can energize the process in this case. An emotional commitment to being rid of it is essential.

You can employ this technique for any kind of discomfort or stress, whether physical, mental, or emotional.

Technique number two: Think about the pain. Yes, think about it. Let your mind, not your emotions, work on this pain. Not with fear but with logical, analytical examination. Or even curiosity. You are concerned about it, of course, yet now be curious, interested in it. Investigate it. Elaine admits this sounds strange. However, it is quite naturally difficult to think and feel at the same time. Stress is an arousal state for the nervous system and the whole body; and just as we cannot be relaxed and tense at the same time, we cannot feel and think clearly, or be emotional and think logically at the same time. One or the other process has to go into the background. So if we are feeling, thinking goes into the background; if we are thinking, feeling goes into the background.

So think about the pain in every way you can. Examine it with your mind. What is it really like? If you were going to describe it to someone, perhaps a doctor, you would have to be very specific. Where exactly is it? Is it closer to the surface deep? Does it feel in the flesh or bone, or in an organ? Is it dull or sharp? Is it hot or cold? And so on ... by the time you've explained all the details to yourself about the pain, you will probably have reduced it if not eliminated it completely.

This works for mental and emotional pain.

Technique number three: This might seem even stranger but there is a scientific basis for its effectiveness. *Do your best to increase the pain*; actually encourage the pain to intensify. Persuading every way you can think of to increase it as much as possible. Talk to it. Say things like, "Come on, you can hurt me more than that!" And mean it! If this sounds paradoxical, considering how much you want to be free of it, and not feel it at all anymore; you are right. For, in fact, there are paradoxical aspects to the nature of the subconscious and its ways of working. This third method works on a very simple principle: the brainstem, the central switchboard to the brain (it is at the base of your skull) that connects it to the body can only process so much information at one time. By forcing the pain to increase, you will be forcing the brainstem to switch it off, to shutdown the communication, because it cannot handle that much.

You will recognize in this echoes of the gate theory which says that when a competing signal reaches a certain strength it will suppress similar or related signals. It is a survival tactic as old as humans themselves, to shut down when things become overwhelming. This is probably why some people feel faint or become unconscious when pain is extreme.

Regardless of scientific support for this technique, you will find that, by employing it, you will be using the built-in system that nature has set up for your benefit. It works very quickly. Elaine reports that the longest amount of time to get the desired result that has been reported to her from people she's taught this technique is about 45 seconds. Most of us can handle intense pain for at least that long, knowing there will be a beneficial result at the end.

You will want a copy of Elaine's amazing book: *The Mind Is Willing*, copyright © 2006 by Elaine Kissel. You can get a copy from: www.elainekissel. com

HERBS

We'll look at some herbs for pain. But I don't want you to think along the same lines as taking medications—just masking the pain and not caring about why you've got it. You still need to be active in seeking health solutions, not just treating symptoms.

However, there are some herbs worth mentioning. They may seem to a layman to be natural, friendly and safe. But don't be naïve: opium is a herb, so are belladonna (deadly poison), hemlock (which was used to put Socrates to death), and aconite (monkshood or wolf's bane).

Treat herbs with the utmost respect and caution and you'll be just fine.

Same with Chinese herbs. These are honored with a long tradition but that doesn't mean they're safe as Mama's apple pie! Be realistic.

Plant pharmacology is very complex and many ingredients are beyond our current knowledge and understanding. Orthodox medical scientists talk about the "active ingredient," as if only one substance in the plant was producing any effect. This is being naïve to the point of stupidity.

Just keep your head, that's all I'm asking. And, as always, seek the advice of a competent professional if you can. The Internet opens up many possibilities today for getting advice at a distance.

Arnica Montana

There are few plant substances I love as much as this kindly herb. It's the perfect answer to soreness, bruising, aches, and even injuries. It contains helenin, an analgesic, as well as anti-inflammatory chemicals. It's easy to take but you can also buy it as a homeopathic remedy at most health food stores. Use 6X or for more chronic pain, 30C.

Arnica is also available in creams and tablets. Apply cream twice daily; use tablets according to package directions.

Comfrey

Comfrey's folk name in Britain is "knit-bone." That tells you what it's good for. Scientific name: *Symphytum officinale* or *Symphytum uplandicum*.

But it's also a useful all-round analgesic, which can benefit injuries and degenerative conditions such as arthritis. Comfrey oil was once popular but it has the potential for causing liver cancer. It's safer to use the cream or ointment and as tea infusions (which is best for broken bones). Tastes awful! Incidentally, don't use *young* comfrey leaves, which contain poisons called pyrrolizidine alkaloids that are carcinogenic.

I found this recipe for comfrey ointment on the Web, from Christine at Slow Living Essentials (she got it from a very old recipe book).

Ingredients:
- 300ml vegetable oil (I used olive, although sunflower is also recommended)
- large handful of comfrey leaves
- 25g-30g beeswax, grated for faster melting

Place as many comfrey leaves as you can cram into a small pot, cover with the chosen oil and simmer over a low heat until the leaves are mushy and the oil has turned green. It was a bit of a guessing process as this was the first ointment I had made. It may be better to do this in a *bain marie* to be sure the oil does not overheat and burn.

The oil is left to cool slightly and then strained. For a stronger oil, this process could be repeated a second and third time if need be.

The grated beeswax is then added to the comfrey oil and placed back over a low heat for a couple of minutes, until the beeswax melts into the oil. Pour the whole into a clean salsa jar and leave uncovered until set. Any residue in the bottom of the pan should be left in there and not added to the jar as this excess moisture will cause the ointment to spoil faster.

Yield: 300ml, with a shelf life of several months.
(www.slowlivingessentials.com)

Oil of Wintergreen

Wintergreen is an analgesic, anti-spasmodic, anti-inflammatory, and anti-rheumatic. It contains methyl salicylate, a direct relative of salicylic acid, the main ingredient in aspirin, so it's not surprising that it is effective as an analgesic.

Did you know that wintergreen essential oil contains 85-99% of methyl salicylate, the same component as aspirin?

Yes, birch and wintergreen were considered the best essential oils for pain before synthetics were made in the early 1920s. The Native Americans used them to combat pain since before we were keeping any records!

Birch and wintergreen are the only plants that naturally contain methyl salicylate. It is documented that these oils have cortisone-like effects that can relieve pain quickly.

Wintergreen is also emotionally warming and soothing. It opens the heart chakra so we are more accepting of ourselves, which is also so important when we are going through any kind of pain.

Birch essential oil is no longer available because of the scarcity of the birch tree. However, wintergreen essential oil is available and is one of my favorite oils to use for a variety of things.

Feverfew

Feverfew (*Tanacetum parthenium*) is a perennial plant belonging to the daisy family that grows in much of Europe, North America and Canada. It has been used in herbal remedies for centuries.

It's famous for headache, especially migraine. A small but competent study published in 2005 demonstrated its efficacy of feverfew as a viable preventative treatment for migraine.

It is available in 60-mg capsules of fresh, powdered leaf (1 to 6 capsules daily), or 25-mg capsules of freeze-dried leaf (2 capsules daily).

You can grow your own in the garden and make feverfew tea—but be warned; it's very bitter and may irritate the mouth. Steep 2 to 8 fresh leaves in boiling water, but do not boil them, since boiling breaks down the active parthenolides.

Feverfew is available as a tincture, but I think the capsules are to be preferred.

Curcumin

Curcumin is one of the pungent active ingredients of turmeric (Curcuma longa), the deep-yellow powder found in virtually every curry dish made in the world. Besides being a culinary delight, several clinical trials have found curcumin to be a notable anti-inflammatory and analgesic compound. Moreover, recent in vitro studies have suggested that curcumin may inhibit COX-2.

Curcumin is being extensively investigated for its anti-cancer and anti-inflammatory properties. It also helps to improve circulation and prevent blood clotting. Turmeric has been used in traditional medicines for easing the pain of sprains, strains, bruises, and joint inflammation, as well as for treating skin and digestive issues.

If you are not already in the habit of enjoying good curries, get to know them. I've been saying for nearly 40 years that Indian curries are mainly good whole food: nothing in the cook pot but vegetables, meats and spices!

You can get ready-made pastes, which are easy to combine with some fried onions and coconut milk. Simmer the chicken, fish, or whatever, with this sauce for a minimum of a half hour and you have a delicious dish!

Just stay away from the naan bread and chapatis and you won't get fat!

Ginger (Zinziber)

Ginger is a natural anti-inflammatory and has been used for thousands of years by the Chinese to cure pain. Ginger helps relieve nausea, arthritis, headaches, menstrual cramps, and muscle soreness.

You can take 1 to 4 grams powdered ginger daily, divided into two to four doses. Or make tea from 1 teaspoon chopped fresh root simmered in a cup of water for about 10 minutes. Let it cool, then strain the water. Or you might prefer ginger tea bags, available in health food stores.

You can also reap relief from pain by applying a ginger compress to the affected area. Grate the root; wrap the ginger in cheesecloth; place it in hot water for 30 seconds; let it cool and place on the affected area for 20 minutes.

Eucommia

Eucommia is a bark (reminiscent of salicylic acid and aspirin). Traditional Chinese herbalists use it for back and joint pain, especially in the hips and knees, and also to strengthen bones, tendons, and ligaments. Eucommia bark helps heal tissue that is slow to mend after an injury or that has been weakened through stress.

Western studies with rats confirm that both the leaves and the bark of eucommia contain a compound that encourages the development of collagen, an important part of connective tissues such as skin, tendons and ligaments. Although it can be used alone, eucommia bark is most often used in combination with other supportive herbs. The only practical way to take eucommia is as a supplement from a licensed provider.

Don't take it with blood pressure medications.

Devil's Claw

Native to southern Africa, devil's claw (Harpagophytum procumbens) gets its name from the tiny hooks that cover its fruit. Historically, devil's claw has been used to treat pain, liver and kidney problems, fever, and malaria. It has also been used in ointments applied to the skin to heal sores, boils, and other skin problems.

Devil's claw was introduced to Europe in the early 1900s, where the dried roots have been used to restore appetite, relieve heartburn, and reduce pain and inflammation.

Today, devil's claw is used to fight inflammation or relieve pain in arthritis, headache, and low back pain. Animal and test tube studies suggest that devil's claw can help fight inflammation, and it is used widely in Germany and France.

The University of Maryland website tells us that several studies have found that taking devil's claw for 8-12 weeks reduces pain and improves physical functioning in people with osteoarthritis of the spine, hip, and knee.

There are also some studies suggesting that devil's claw may help relieve low back and neck pain. Patients who took devil's claw every day for a month said they had less pain and needed fewer painkillers than those who took placebo.

It has other uses. Many professional herbalists suggest devil's claw to treat upset stomach, loss of appetite, headaches, allergies, and fever. Topical preparations of devil's claw are also applied to the skin to heal sores, ulcers, boils, and skin lesions.

Capsaicin

Capsaicin is the ingredient found in different types of hot peppers, such as cayenne, that makes the peppers spicy hot. You can eat it in raw or cooked peppers or as a dried powder, which you can add to food or drinks. It also is available as a dietary supplement and in topical creams that you apply to your skin.

Capsaicin works by first stimulating and then decreasing the intensity of pain signals in the body. Although pain may at first increase, it usually decreases after the first use (remember the pain gating theory, which says that excess signals will shut down the perception of pain).

As a skin preparation it can be used for:

- Pain disorders, including pain after surgery.
- Nervous system problems, such as diabetic neuropathy, trigeminal neuralgia, and post-herpetic neuralgia (bad pains after shingles).
- Cluster headaches.
- Joint problems, such as osteoarthritis and rheumatoid arthritis.
- Skin conditions, such as psoriasis.
- Mouth sores due to chemotherapy or radiation (Traumeel is better, page 53).

In general, you use creams containing capsaicin for pain relief. You can put the creams on your skin up to four times a day.

Wash your hands thoroughly after each use to avoid getting the cream in your eyes or on other moist mucous membranes, where it can cause a burning sensation. Do not use the cream on areas of broken skin; it will hurt like hell!

Peppermint

Peppermint (*Mentha piperita*) is a famous antispasmodic for digestive cramps. It is often used as the oil. A 1994 study showed that peppermint essential oil was effective at blocking channels that transmit pain signals. It's powerful stuff.

Germany's Commission E authorizes use of oral peppermint oil for treating colicky pain in the digestive tract of adults (peppermint oil shouldn't be used for colic in newborn babies, as it can cause jaundice).

Several double-blind studies of individuals with irritable bowel syndrome demonstrate that peppermint can significantly relieve painful abdominal cramps, bloating, and flatulence. In the largest study, reported in the *Journal of Gastroenterology*, researchers administered either enteric-coated peppermint oil or a placebo to 110 individuals three to four times daily, 15 to 30 minutes before meals, for four weeks. The study found peppermint significantly reduced abdominal discomfort.

For mild stomach discomfort, try a tea from fresh or dried peppermint leaves.

For something tougher, use the oil, which is concentrated. The menthol in peppermint relaxes the muscles. Its antispasmodic and analgesic effects also can help relieve headaches, possibly including migraines, when applied to the forehead or temples—dilute about 3 drops of essential oil in 1 tablespoon of vegetable oil.

Oil Of Cloves

Clove (*Syzygium aromaticum*) is great for tooth pain. It's a very strong oil. Just rub it into the gums near the site of pain. It can be very soothing.

Licorice root (*Glycyrrhiza glabra*) has made it onto the orthodox medicine stage, just in my lifetime. It's no longer just flavored goo for kids' stickjaw; it's a pharmaceutical!

Licorice contains 9 anesthetic compounds, 10 analgesic compounds, and 20 anti-inflammatory compounds. Small wonder it's good for pain. We used to buy twigs of the root; you can fray the end like a brush and clean your teeth while chewing it!

To make tea, simmer about 2 teaspoons of dried root in a cup of water for 15 minutes; strain. Do not take licorice if you have high blood pressure, heart conditions, diabetes, kidney disease, or glaucoma.

Essential Oil Therapy

Essential oils are a whole class of successful medicinal treatments and have many health applications. Aromatherapy (section 18) is a related discipline but not totally interchangeable. There are over 60 different essential oils for pain that have analgesic properties.

Essential, by the way, does not mean necessary or have-to-have; it means from essences (smells). These remedies all comes from flavored and highly scented plant oils, like rosemary, lavender, and oregano.

Mixtures

You can also get proprietary mixtures of oils, such as PanAway Essential Oil Blend™. Documented uses for PanAway Essential Oil include headaches, a natural anti-inflammatory, relieves pain from rheumatism and arthritis, bone pain, circulation, sprains, muscle spasms and injuries. This formula is just an example, but it contains four different essential oils.

- Peppermint essential oil is cooling to the skin. It blocks pain and enhances the other effects of the oils.
- Wintergreen essential oil (Gaultheria procumbens) is warming. It contains methyl salicylate and has a cortisone-like effect that reduces pain and inflammation from muscles, and joints.
- Helichrysum essential oil (Helichrysum italicum) is a powerful natural anti-inflammatory. It also improves circulation and may help cleanse the blood.
- Clove essential oil (Syzygium aromaticum) has anti-inflammatory, antiseptic, anesthetic, and anti-infectious properties! That's why clove essential oil is so powerful for arthritis and rheumatism.

See page 4 for the theory that a lot of arthritis condition may turn out to be bacterial infections in nature.

Soothing the State of Mind

Look again at the three dimensions of pain in the introduction (page 6). One of them is definitely the psychological component, not just the physical signals. So essential oils therapy, administered by a knowledgeable expert, is bound to be superior to merely blocking the nerve sensations, as analgesics do.

So pain sufferers may derive much more benefit from herbs with calming or sedative properties, such as lavender (Lavandula angustifolia), chamomile (Matricaria recutita), or valerian (Valeriana officinalis).

How To

All essential oils are used in a similar way, though individual practitioners have their own ways.

Use diluted, 50:50 dilution (one part essential oil to one part of a vegetable oil). Then:

- Apply several drops (2-4) on location to muscles or injury
- Apply to temples for headache
- Apply to chakras/vitaflex points
- Apply as compress on spine
- Directly inhale, or use
- Your candle diffuser

For more helpful suggestions, see also section 31 "Anti-Inflammatory Supplements"

CANNABIS (POT, HASHISH, MARIJUANA, SHIT, DRAW, WEED...)

I'm including this topic here, as separate from "drugs" for pain (section 2), by which I intended to mean medical drugs. Although "medical marijuana" is now a watchword and rallying cry, there are plenty of people who would stop short of considering it a medically-approved substance, whatever national and federal laws decide.

However, evidence is fairly conclusive that cannabinoids substantially relieve pain (the active ingredients in marijuana), according to a detailed 1999 report by *The Institute of Medicine* [Philippe Lucas (January 2012). "It can't hurt to ask; a patient-centered quality of service assessment of health Canada's medical cannabis policy and program". Harm Reduct J 9 (2): 2.]

If nothing else is coming your way that helps with pain, you may wish to consider it. I just don't want you to approach it in ignorance, so here we go...

Chronic pain is one of the most commonly cited reasons for the use of medical marijuana. It rose to prominence for the relief of suffering in terminal cancer cases and grew from there. A 2012 Canadian survey of participants in their medical marijuana program found that 84% of respondents reported using medical marijuana for the management of pain.["Medical Marijuana and Chronic Pain". www.truthonpot.com. TruthOnPot.com. 11 March 2013. Retrieved 28 April 2013]

The principal psychoactive constituent of cannabis is called tetrahydrocannabinol (THC). It is one of over 480 compounds found in the Cannabis plant, including at least 84 other cannabinoids, such as cannabidiol (CBD), cannabinol (CBN), tetrahydrocannabivarin (THCV) and cannabigerol (CBG).

In a 2013 review study published in *Fundamental & Clinical Pharmacology*, various studies were cited in demonstrating that cannabinoids exhibit comparable effectiveness to opioids in models of acute pain and even greater effectiveness in models of chronic pain.[31]

Scientists from Imperial College London found that Cannador, another cannabis plant extract, effectively relieved pain after major surgery. They reported their findings in the journal *Anesthesiology*.

Researchers from McGill University Health Centre (MUHC) and McGill University reported in CMAJ in 2010 that patients with chronic neuropathic pain experienced pain relief, improved mood and better quality sleep after smoking cannabis.

In January 2017, the National Academies of Science published an exhaustive review of the scientific literature and found that one of the most promising areas in medical cannabis is for the treatment of chronic pain. [The Health Effects of Cannabis and Cannabinoids: The Current State of Evidence and Recommendations for Research. Released Jan 12th 2017]

However, researchers from Oxford University's Centre for Functional Magnetic Resonance Imaging of the Brain (FMRIB) found no evidence that THC tablets reduced the pain intensity induced by 1% capsaicin cream (hot chillie). It simply made it more bearable.

In this new study, brain imaging shows little reduction in the brain regions that code for the sensation of pain, which is what we tend to see with drugs like opiates. Instead cannabis appears to mainly affect the emotional reaction to pain in a highly variable way. According to researchers, some people responded really well, others not at all, or even poorly.

In other words, the study revealed new information about the neural basis of cannabis-induced pain relief. Cannabis does not seem to act like a conventional pain medicine.

Whatever the outcome of emergent laws, legislation cannot make smoking it a clean, healthy habit.

The propaganda position is that marijuana is harmless, a position with which I take strong exception. Unwanted side-effects can include a decrease in short-term memory, impaired motor skills (making driving while buzzed totally unsafe), reddening of the eyes and feelings of paranoia or anxiety.

It should never be used by persons with a history of schizoid symptoms and those with a family history of mental illness should be cautious in the extreme.

Cannabis, like tobacco, has lots of chemical, which render long-term or heavy use a danger for lung disease and possibly cancer. The risk is greater because cannabis is often mixed with tobacco and smoked without a filter.

A reduction in sperm count for men and suppressed ovulation in women have been reported with frequent use of cannabis. Both can markedly affect fertility.

Whether or not there are some medical benefits to this substance, there are clear and considerable dangers which, of course, are conveniently overlooked or sidelined by those who are engaged in what I consider profiteering and legalized drug-pushing.

However, times are clearly changing and what I think will soon be largely irrelevant. But having seen the worst of the results of cannabis abuse, I am not sanguine as to its frequent use and certainly do not encourage it if there is a possibility of a full resolution to the pain problem. Terminal cases, maybe.

One thing I will concede:

Cannabidiol (CBD) Helps Break Opioid Addictions

First of its kind study on mice shows undeniable evidence that cannabis extract cannabidiol (CBD) can cure deadly opioid addiction.

Scientists have shown that CBD actually blocks the opioid receptor in the brain, leaving no more doubt that cannabis makes sense as a treatment for opioid addiction.

As the opioid epidemic rages on, those professing to seek "solutions" are willfully ignoring one of the most promising treatments – cannabidiol. When the Comprehensive Addiction & Recovery Act (CARA) was being debated in 2016, amendments to study medical cannabis were stripped out.

This happened despite the government's own National Institutes of Health stating, "Medical marijuana products may have a role in reducing the use of opioids needed to control pain."

Example: a study published in JAMA 2014, compared opioid death rates in states with liberalized marijuana laws with those that legalized in later. [JAMA Intern Med. 2014;174(10):1668-1673. doi:10.1001/jamainternmed.2014.4005]

"Three states (California, Oregon, and Washington) had medical cannabis laws effective prior to 1999. Ten states (Alaska, Colorado, Hawaii, Maine, Michigan, Montana, Nevada, New Mexico, Rhode Island, and Vermont) enacted medical cannabis laws between 1999 and 2010. States with medical cannabis laws had a 24.8% lower mean annual opioid overdose mortality rate…compared with states without medical cannabis laws. Examination of the association between medical cannabis laws and opioid analgesic overdose mortality in each year after implementation of the law showed that such laws were associated with a lower rate of overdose mortality that generally strengthened over time. In secondary analyses, the findings remained similar."

A 2016 study surveying 473 adults showed that 80 percent of cannabis users give up prescription pills. [Lucas, P., Walsh, Z., Crosby, K., Callaway, R., Belle-Isle, L., Kay, R., Capler, R., and Holtzman, S. (2016) Substituting cannabis for prescription drugs, alcohol and other substances among medical cannabis patients: The impact of contextual factors. Drug Alcohol Rev, 35: 326–333. doi: 10.1111/dar.12323]

Whereas the use of a cannabis derivative may have some people frowning, it is unquestionably better and safer than taking opioids.

But all of this falls on deaf ears to those in the pockets of Big Pharma, which is largely to blame for getting America hooked on opioids, as described in a Harvard analysis. They don't want the addiction (and overdose) epidemic to end.

MASSAGE AND AROMATHERAPY

In a star rating system, this would probably be a one-star treatment, whereas SCENAR, homotoxicology or the anti-inflammatory diet would rate four stars. Of course, proponents are enthusiastic and for them it means lots of repeat business. Basically, I consider it pleasant and helpful but very shallow. It's not curative. Restoring health is always the target, not palliative symptomatic treatment.

That said, you are promised a comprehensive guide to pain control, so let's take a look.

Massage

Massage is well known to relieve temporary pain, such as that due to excessive physical activity and it is great to experience, after a sports game or a tough hike!

On a deeper level, therapeutic massage, which can include variants such as shiatsu and tui na, may be able to soothe troubled tissues long enough to affect at least some healing. As I wrote in the section on backache (page 155), oftentimes the real persistent pain comes from tension and muscle spasm, more in anticipation of pain than its actual intensity.

There is some interesting science to all this…

Each collagen molecule is a strong dipole, i.e., it has two oppositely charged ends. The head is the bigger part and it has a slightly larger positive charge, while the tail is smaller and it has a slightly smaller negative charge. Thus the overall charge of each collagen molecule is positive.

Collagen molecules unite together to form different anatomical structures (tendons, ligaments, bones, structural frame of the inner organs, etc.). All collagen molecules in combination with other electrically active proteins generate a so-called, fixed electric charge of each organ and tissue.

Thus, the fixed electric charge is a cumulative charge of all electrically active molecules in the area. Even under normal conditions this charge constantly changes as a result of the individual person's physical activity, diet, level of stress, etc. Despite these constant fluctuations, changes in the fixed electric charge stay within the physiological range assigned to this particular tissue.

The situation changes dramatically if the soft tissue or inner organ is traumatized or has developed inflammation, etc. The fixed electric charge within the affected area immediately changes its normal value as a result of the pathological process.

Any inflammation or trauma of the soft tissue increases the positive fixed electric charge and the collagen fibers are one of the major contributors to this process. Swelling, rupture, and twisting of the normal collagen fibers greatly contribute to the increase of the positive fixed charge in the soft tissue. The healing process after initial trauma or inflammation is always accompanied by slow restoration of the fixed electric charge in the affected area.

During the massage, external mechanical stimuli in form of repeated application of massage strokes deform the collagen molecules and generate the piezoelectricity that increases the negative fixed electric charge. As we discussed above, the negative electric charge has the greatest impact on the proliferation, growth, and regeneration of the tissue.

Also, the increase of the negative charge in the affected area is the critical factor in the correct alignment of the pro-collagen fibers before their maturation into the fully developed collagen fibers. The delay of this process slows the local healing. Thus the restoration of the fixed electric charge is a critically important process in reducing the tension in the soft tissue and eliminating the physical and even mental stress. At the same time, it is an equally important component in speeding up the healing process.

The concept of piezoelectricity gives the practitioners a lot of important clinical tools to apply therapy correctly and optimize the outcomes of the treatment. For example, the study conducted by Shamos and Lavine in 1967 showed that human skin exhibits the largest piezoelectrical potentials if the mechanical stimuli are applied at under a 45-degree angle. This is a very important practical recommendation, as the massage practitioner needs to generate the greatest number of piezo-electrical potentials during the treatment.

Modern technology allows scientists to measure the piezoelectrical properties even within a single collagen fiber. In their recent study, Minary-Jolandan and Yu (2009) showed that single collagen fiber is able to generate a piezoelectric coefficient of 1 pm V(-1) and the summation of piezoelectrical charges generated by each collagen fiber allow the entire tendon to generate electric potential up to tens of millivolts, depending upon the size of the tendon. The authors of this study strongly reinforced the previously mentioned publication of Shamos and Lavine, who found that only shear deformation of the collagen fibers triggers the piezoelectrical effect. Thus the angle of the application of the pressure during the massage strokes (45 degrees is the most preferable) is a critical factor in the generation of the piezoelectricity and normalization of the electrophysiological properties of the soft tissue.

A very important article for massage practitioners was published in 1977 by one of the most respected scientific authorities in the field of bioelectricity, Professor B. Lipinski, MD. Using his experimental data, he formulated the theory that links the therapeutic effect of soft tissue manipulations, acupuncture, hatha yoga, and the action of negatively charged air ions with piezoelectrical properties of the biological tissue.

According to this theory, proteins, mucopolysaccahrides, nucleic acids, etc., which compose all tissue of our body are able to generate piezo-electricity. Thus, these substances have the ability to transfer the externally applied mechanical energy (e.g., by massage strokes) into electric energy inside the soft tissue.

The author showed that stimulation of the soft tissue in the special areas on the body produces the electric current. This piezoelectrically-induced current activates the healing processes in the stimulated area, and it is able to flow "towards the internal organs along the semiconductive channels of biological micromolecules."

Hence, every time you apply mechanical pressure to the soft tissue in the form of massage strokes, you actively produce the electric current in these tissues, and it has enormous healing potential on the cellular, tissue, and organ levels. This electric current is able to travel to the distant parts of the body, including the inner organs, and normalize their function.

The healing impact of the massage treatment is directly correlated with the total amount of piezoelectrical potentials the practitioner need to generate during the therapy. If the practitioner doesn't use correct tools and tips (e.g., angle of the strokes, speed of the strokes, greater variety of massage techniques, etc.) he or she greatly diminishes the healing outcomes of the treatment and undermines his or her efforts and practice.

Aromatherapy

Recent studies corroborate the use of aromatherapy for pain relief. "Aromatherapy is effective because it works directly on the amygdala, the brain's emotional center," says Mehmet Oz, MD, professor of surgery at Columbia University Medical Center in New York City. "This has important consequences because the thinking part of the brain can't inhibit the effects of the scent, meaning you feel them instantaneously." Of the many uses of aromatherapy, pain relief is only one; anxiety reduction and rejuvenation are other common objectives.

Well, if Dr. Oz says it works, who am I to argue?

Dr. Oz, a cardiovascular surgeon, studied aromatherapy to find alternative methods to expedite recovery time and reduce anxiety in heart patients. Dr. Oz and his collaborator, clinical aromatherapist Jane Buckle, PhD, recommend using 15 drops of an essential oil, such as lavender, chamomile or eucalyptus, diluted with 1 oz. (2 Tbsp.) of a "carrier" or neutral oil, such as almond, avocado or jojoba, dabbed directly on the skin. This means you literally have scented relief on you when you need it.

Clinical aromatherapists commonly use lavender, peppermint, chamomile, and damask rose oils for pain relief and relaxation. A report from Nursing Clinics of North America says that massage with lavender relieves pain and enhances the effect of orthodox pain medication.

Lavender and chamomile oils are gentle enough to be used with children and can be used in blends. Both oils contain anti-inflammatory and antispasmodic chemicals, and exert sedative, calming action. Rose essential oil contains pain-reducing eugenol, cinnamaldehyde, and geraniol.

Maybe hints of the garden also help calm and sooth patients in pain or distress?

You can find more suggested essential oils for all kinds of pain, in the section on Herbs (section 16).

Smell Is Key

Alan Hirsch, MD, neurologist at the Smell and Taste Treatment and Research Foundation in Chicago, believes you don't have to limit yourself to essential oils. Limiting the length of your exposure to certain scents, however, will ensure they remain effective. "Short-term exposure is key because people stop responding to scents after a few minutes," he says.

To use aromatherapy for pain, relaxation, and rejuvenation, Drs. Hirsch and Oz recommend trying these scents.

Relax: vanilla. In the Columbia University Medical Center study, subjects who smelled vanilla while completing stress tests had more stable heart rates and blood pressure readings than those who took the tests in an unscented environment.

Try placing a few drops of vanilla extract onto a handkerchief and carry it with you throughout the day.

Recharge: peppermint, jasmine, citrus. These scents make you feel more awake. "Even though these scents are pleasant, they act as mild irritants and the effect is similar to that of smelling salts," explains Dr. Hirsch.

Try sprinkling a few drops of the essential oil of your choice in a candle diffuser, or dilute two drops in 1 tsp. of avocado or almond oil, then rub it onto the back of your hand.

Relieve: Green apple. "We found that the smell of green apples reduced the severity and duration of migraine headache pain and may have a similar effect on joint pain," says Dr. Hirsch. "The scent seems to reduce muscle contractions, which are the main cause of pain in migraines."

[SOURCE: Arthritis Foundation (www.arthritistoday.org)]

BIOELECTRIC THERAPY

Electronic Pain Management Devices

The classic and well-established device of this type is the TENS unit. "TENS" stands for transcutaneous electrical nerve stimulation.

There are other units you may care to investigate, such as the MicroAce device and the Gyrotonic.

In TENS therapy for pain management, a small, battery-operated device delivers low-voltage electrical current through the skin via electrodes placed near the source of pain. The electricity from the electrodes stimulates nerves in the affected area and sends signals to the brain that block normal pain perception. TENS is not painful and may be effective therapy to mask pain such as diabetic neuropathy.

However, TENS for chronic low back pain is now said to be not very effective and the American Academy of Neurology (AAN) recommends against it.

TENS, by definition, covers the complete range of transcutaneously applied currents used for nerve excitation, although the term is often used with a more restrictive intent, namely to describe the kind of pulses produced by portable stimulators used to treat pain. The unit is usually connected to the skin using two or more electrodes. A typical battery-operated TENS unit is able to modulate pulse width, frequency, and intensity. Generally TENS is applied at high frequency (>50 Hz) with an intensity below motor contraction (sensory intensity) or low frequency (<10 Hz) with an intensity that produces motor contraction. [Wiki]

The benefit of TENS for pain is controversial. It was originally thought to work via the pain gating mechanism; that is, TENS overwhelms the gating system, so that it becomes refractory and so can no longer transmit pain signals.

The worry now is that TENS actually damages the nerves and the failure to function may become permanent, which is not as beneficial as you might think (see introduction, page 2, for notes on the *value* of pain).

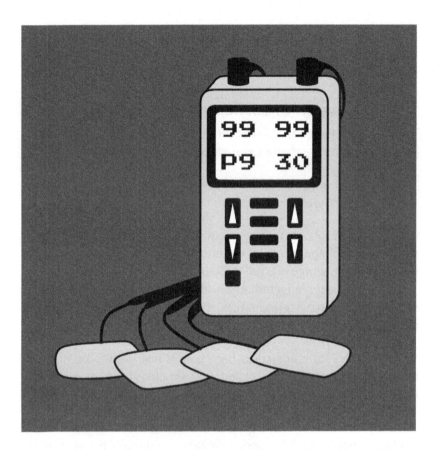

Outcomes

One review from 2007 felt that the evidence supports a benefit in chronic musculoskeletal pain, while another review from the Cochrane Collaboration in 2008 deemed the evidence of poor quality and thus no conclusions were possible regarding chronic pain. Results from a task force on neck pain, in 2008, found no clinically significant benefit to TENS for the treatment of neck pain when compared to placebo treatment. [Haldeman S, Carroll L, Cassidy JD, Schubert J, Nygren Å. The bone and joint decade 2000–2010 task force on neck pain and its associated disorders. *Spine* 33 (4 Suppl): S5–S7.]

A 2010 review did not find evidence to support the use of TENS for chronic low back pain. There is tentative evidence that it may be useful for painful diabetic neuropathy. [Dubinsky R M, Miyasaki J. Assessment: Efficacy of transcutaneous electric nerve stimulation in the treatment of pain in neurologic disorders (an evidence-based review): Report of the Therapeutics and Technology Assessment Subcommittee of the American Academy of Neurology. *Neurology*. 2009; 74(2): 173–176.]

Nevertheless, proponents continue to advocate its effectiveness. Just bear in mind the vested interest of practitioners who have bought a TENS device!

Note: Today many people confuse TENS with electro muscle stimulation (EMS). EMS and TENS devices look similar, with both using long electric lead wires and electrodes. TENS is for blocking pain, where EMS is for stimulating muscles. Some devices combine both modalities.

Surgical Intervention Techniques

This is not to be confused with radiofrequency discal nucleoplasty, which is a surgical procedure that utilizes a radio frequency probe instead of heating wire to disintegrate a small portion of the intervertebral disc material. The result of this intervention is a partial decompression of the disc, which may help relieve pain caused by bulging discs pressing on nearby spinal nerve roots.

Spinal cord stimulation (SCS) system is a hybrid system comprising implanted electrodes in the spine and an external control unit. It uses electrical stimulation to block the pain pathways to the brain that travel through the spinal cord. SCS has also been known to decrease spasticity. An initial trial is needed to see if effective results can be achieved. If the trial is successful, a permanent system may be implanted. The user has the ability to keep the system on permanently or as needed.

Intradiscal electrothermal therapy (IDET) is a treatment option for people with low back pain resulting from intervertebral disc problems.

Intervertebral discs act as cushions between the vertebrae. Sometimes the discs can become damaged and swell, causing pain. IDET uses heat to modify the nerve fibers of a spinal disc and to destroy pain receptors in the area. In this procedure, a wire called an electrothermal catheter is placed through an incision in the disc. An electrical current passes through the wire, heating a small outer portion of the disc to a temperature of 90 degrees Celsius. IDET is performed as an outpatient procedure while the patient is awake and under local anesthesia.

These are far from "natural" or self-help pain therapies and I am definitely NOT supporting them. I mention them only for disambiguation (clarity).

TENS and PENS units

- Algotech Ltd. - Providing a neurostimulation PENS Therapy for chronic pain. (http://www.algotec-ltd.com)
- Axelgaard - Their PALS Electrodes have become the world-wide brand of neurostimulation electrode. (http://www.axelgaard.com)
- Axiobionics, LLC - Wearable therapies are custom-built external electrical stimulation systems. (http://www.wearabletherapy.com
- Biowave - They designed three pain therapy devices, all using percutaneous neuromodulation therapy therapeutic electrical signal into deep tissue: Deepwave, Homewave and Sportswave. (http://www.biowave.com)
- Care Rehab - They offer TENS units for the treatment of pain. (http://www.carerehab.com/tens.html)
- Dynatronics - Providing self-administered TENS devices to manage post-traumatic or post-surgical pain. (http://www.dynatronics.com)
- Electronmedical Products International - Alpha-Stim device treats pain and stress-related disorders with a proven, safe, effective non-drug approach. (http://www.alpha-stim.com)
- Empi, Inc. - Empi's extensive line of rehabilitation products offer solutions for a variety of health care needs, including pain control options. (http://www.djoglobal.com/our-brands/empi)
- Medical Science Products - Specializing in non-invasive electrotherapy devices. (http://www.medsciencepro.com)
- NeuroMetrix - Offering the SENSUS device focusing on treatment for painful diabetic neuropathy. http://www.neurometrix.com/
- Neurotech - Wearable TENS units for the treatment of chronic pain include Baxolve XP, Aviva TENS XP and Recovery Back devices. (http://www.neurotechgroup.com/us/go/product-categories/pain-management)
- RS Medical - Offering pain and function solution stimulators to treat painful muscle conditions and to treat persistent back and neck pain. (http://www.rsmedical.com)

- SPR Therapeutics - Offering a peripheral nerve stimulation system for shoulder pain. (http://www.sprtherapeutics.com)

Others:

- Anodyne Therapy - Anodyne® Infrared Therapy Systems are medical devices that are indicated to increase circulation and reduce pain, stiffness, and muscle spasm. (http://www. anodynetherapy.com)
- Neuros Medical - Developing nerve block technology for chronic pain. (http://www.neurosmedical.com)

Always insist on a trial period, if you can get one.

You might do better financially to shop for one at Amazon.com or OverStock.com.

See also: SCENAR and Avazzia, section 12

BIOFEEDBACK

Most people today have at least heard of the biofeedback principle. It relates mainly to involuntary functions in the body. With things we can control voluntarily, we simply do as we wish.

But certain body functions, like heart rate and blood pressure, we can't immediately control. However, we can eventually learn to regulate them, if we get some kind of feedback to tell us which way things are going.

Take heart rate: if you heard a soft whine that went lower and lower in tone as your heart rate dropped, you could hear the changes. Then you simply tweak your mental state, until you find out what you need to do to get that heart rate lower.

Biofeedback, then, is simply the signaling device that tells you what is happening to your physiology. After a short time, you can take control, with the feedback to help you.

Peripheral Temperature

Cold hands and feet, sweaty palms, are symptoms of stress and anxiety. The "peripheral temperature," as it's called, is a good measure of how relaxed you are. Cold and sweaty, of course, denotes a lower peripheral temperature (clammy). The opposite is a nice warm periphery, showing how calm you are!

For a few dollars, you can buy a digital thermometer that measures skin temperature. You can attach the electrode to a finger and read off the temperature scale.

If you can learn to relax, you will see your peripheral temperature rise. It's like a reward; the calmer you feel, the more the temperature at your finger ends will rise.

So you will quickly appreciate why this approach is called "biofeedback." Something—some electrical sensor with sound or visual signal—is present, to tell you how you are doing. This feedback helps you focus on making subtle changes in your body, such as relaxing certain muscles, to achieve the results you want. That can include reducing pain.

In essence, biofeedback gives you the power to use your thoughts to control your body, often to help with a health condition or physical performance. Biofeedback is most commonly used as a relaxation technique.

Biofeedback has a number of advantages:

- It's noninvasive.
- It may reduce medications (running alongside) or eliminate the need for medications.
- It can be used where a patient can't tolerate medications.
- It may be useful during pregnancy, when medications are inappropriate.
- It helps people take charge of their own health.

Therapy

Biofeedback is something you can do for yourself. However, it's highly recommended to get professional help at first. While you are new to it and don't know what to expect, the guidance of an expert will always be welcome.

To find a biofeedback therapist, start by asking your doctor or another health professional with knowledge of biofeedback therapy to recommend someone who has experience treating your condition. Many biofeedback therapists are licensed in another area of health care, such as nursing or physical therapy, and might work under the guidance of a doctor. But state laws regulating biofeedback practitioners vary. Some biofeedback therapists choose to become certified to show their extra training and experience in the practice.

Ask a potential biofeedback therapist questions before starting treatment, such as:

- Are you licensed, certified, or registered?
- If you aren't licensed, are you working under the supervision of a licensed health care professional?

- What is your training and experience?
- Do you have experience providing feedback for my condition?
- How many biofeedback sessions do you think I'll need?
- What's the cost, and is it covered by health insurance?

During a biofeedback session, a therapist attaches electrical sensors to different parts of your body. These sensors monitor your body's physiological state, such as brain waves, skin temperature, or muscle tension. This information is fed back to you via cues, such as a beeping sound or a flashing light. The feedback teaches you to change or control your body's physiological reactions by changing your thoughts, emotions, or behavior. In turn, this can help the condition for which you sought treatment.

For instance, biofeedback can pinpoint tense muscles that are causing back pain spasm or headaches. When the spasm vanishes, it will help relieve the discomfort of conditions like low back pain, abdominal pain, temporomandibular joint disorders (TMJ), and fibromyalgia. For pain relief, biofeedback can benefit people of all ages, from children to older adults.

Headaches are particularly well served. Muscle tension and stress can trigger migraines and other types of headaches and can make headache symptoms worse. There is good evidence that biofeedback therapy can relax muscles and ease stress to reduce both the frequency and severity of headaches.

The ultimate goal with biofeedback is to learn to use these techniques at home on your own.

A typical biofeedback session lasts 30 to 60 minutes. The length and number of sessions are determined by your condition and how quickly you learn to control your physical responses. You may need a series of 10 sessions or as many as 50, which can make it more expensive and time-consuming.

Types of Biofeedback

Your therapist may use several different biofeedback techniques. Determining the technique that's right for you depends on your health problems and goals. Biofeedback techniques include:

- Electromyography (EMG) biofeedback. This type gives

you information about your body's muscle tension so that you can practice relaxation. It may be used for back pain, headaches, anxiety disorders, muscle retraining after injury, and incontinence.

- Temperature (thermal) biofeedback. Skin contact sensors attached to your fingers or feet measure your skin temperature. Because your temperature often drops when you're under stress, a low reading can prompt you to begin relaxation techniques. This type can be used for headache and Raynaud's syndrome.

- Galvanic skin response training. Sensors measure the activity of your sweat glands and the amount of perspiration on your skin, alerting you to anxiety. This measures sweating and can be used for pain and anxiety. We go far deeper with this type of device in my self-help specialty Supernoetics™; however, fuller explanations are inappropriate here.

- Heart rate variability biofeedback. This type of biofeedback helps you control your heart rate in an effort to improve blood pressure, lung function, and stress and anxiety. Heartmath (www.heartmath.com) has an excellent reputation for this type of device.

- Neurofeedback or electroencephalography (EEG). This measures brain waves. It can help significantly with chronic pain that is refractory to analgesics. The majority of users benefit and are satisfied with the treatment. [Appl Psychophysiol Biofeedback. 2013 Jun; 38(2): 101-8. doi: 10.1007/s10484-013-9214-9.]

Home Treatment Devices

A growing number of biofeedback devices and programs are being marketed for home use. Some of these are hand-held portable devices, while others connect to your computer. You can try different devices until you find one that works for you, or ask your doctor for advice. Check with your health insurance company to see what costs, if any, associated with biofeedback devices are covered.

Be aware that some products marketed as biofeedback devices may not be, and that not all biofeedback practitioners are reputable. If a manufacturer or biofeedback practitioner makes claims that their biofeedback device can assess your organs for disease, find impurities in your blood, cure your condition or send signals into your body, or any other weird kind of woo-woo sounding claims, check with your doctor before using it, as it may not be legitimate.

Experts aren't entirely sure how biofeedback works. But if biofeedback is successful for you, it may help you control symptoms of your condition or reduce the amount of medication you take. Eventually, you can practice the biofeedback techniques you learn on your own. You may need to continue with standard treatment for your condition, though.

On the downside, learning biofeedback can take a lot of time and, if it's not covered by your health insurance, it can be personally expensive. In some cases, biofeedback may be no more effective than other simpler, less expensive relaxation techniques, such as yoga.

BINAURAL BEATS AND BEYOND

This book contains nothing, if not dramatic and very unusual methods for pain control. The next modality may just be the strangest. But it's also one of the most delightful and effective.

It begins with what we call brain entrainment. Most people have heard of binaural beats—playing different frequency sounds to the right and left ear, causing the brain to tune to the difference between the frequencies and synchronizing both hemispheres to that.

For example, if you play 440 Hertz to the right ear and 444 Hertz to the left ear, the brain soon begins to resonate at 4 Hertz (the difference). It so happens that this brainwave frequency is one that we call *theta* (4 – 8 Hertz) and is characteristic of dream and trance states. So what happens? The person listening to these "binaural" (2-sound) beats begins to drift off into a dreamy trance-like state!

Other brainwave frequencies are delta (2 -3 Hertz), which characterizes sleep and unconsciousness; that's good for analgesia, by the way. Alpha means frequencies in the range 9 – 13 Hertz. That's associated with lightly meditative states; somewhat internalized but not "out of it," by any means.

Finally, there is beta frequency (15 -25 hertz) and high beta (over 25 Hertz). These highly active brainwaves appear when the individual is wide awake and alert. In fact at 35 Hertz the person would be getting seriously jittery and over-stimulated, like drinking far too much caffeinated coffee!

So what?

Well, as I explained, we can deliberately create these states in the brain, using the difference in frequency between the two ears. Even more importantly, the two halves of the brain begin to resonate together, at the same frequency. We call this brain integration. It's a slightly non-natural state, meaning it doesn't usually happen. But it's very powerful when it does.

Mental performance is significantly enhanced and that has been found to improve all sorts of abilities: more sleep, faster learning, improved memory, lowers blood pressure, blows away migraine and headaches, relaxes and lowers stress, and helps generate serotonin, the "happy" neuropeptide, which in turn creates a feeling of well-being that can last for several days.

Robert Monroe, one of the pioneers in this field, reported that inducing brain wave patterns through the creation of binaural beats had wide range of effects, including "focusing of attention, suggestibility, problem solving, creativity, memory, and learning...sleep induction, pain control...and enhanced learning..."

Dr. Margaret Patterson, in collaboration with biochemist Dr. Ifor Capel at the Marie Curie Cancer Memorial Foundation Research Department in Surrey, England, has shown that certain frequencies in the brain dramatically speed up production of a variety of neurotransmitters. For instance, a 10 Hz (alpha) signal boosts the production and turnover rate of serotonin, a chemical messenger that increases relaxation and eases pain.

In fact, it's been shown using brain scans in scientific tests that just 7 minutes of brain entrainment can replicate the mind power results of 30 years of meditation!

Photic Driving or Frequency Following

Another way to entrain brain frequencies is with apparatus to create flickering lights. If light is shone into the eyes which varies or "flickers" at around 4 -5 Hertz, it will create a dreamy relaxed theta state.

I have speculated elsewhere that this is why sitting by a log fire can be so soporific. Yellow-tongue flames typically flicker at about 4 -5 Hertz; staring into them we relax and eventually drift off into a trance. It could be carbon monoxide poisoning, of course! But this happens even in the outdoors, around a campfire. No, I'm sure the flicker-following effect, as it's called, is the real reason a blazing fire makes us drowsy.

Actually, the effect of flickering lights was studied long before binaural beats technology, which came about only through Sony and Panasonic small stereo devices (it has to be stereo, to be a different frequency in each ear).

In 1899, Pierre Marie Félix Janet (1859 - 1945) a French physician, psychiatrist, and philosopher, reported noticing a change in the mental state in some of his patients after being subjected to entrainment. They experienced decreasing tension and hysteria as well as increasing relaxation when he exposed them to flickering light created by a rotating strobe-wheel illuminated by a kerosene lantern behind it.

As far as history records it, this is probably the first known clinical application of brainwave entrainment. Since then, the effect has been repeated and described in scientific papers many times.

We call this the "flicker following" effect or "photic driving." It is NOT the same as strobe lighting.

Pain Control

You want to know about pain relief. In broad terms, a theta state will give that sense of the dreamy state of mind that characterizes the opiates. It's been said that it's not so much analgesic as detaching a person from the pain.

Delta states are better at eliminating pain because delta is the equivalent of sleep or unconsciousness.

In 1988, Dr. Normal Shealy tested photic stimulation devices on more than 5,000 patients suffering from chronic pain and stress, using photic driving. A more detailed analysis of 92 of the patients indicated that 88 obtained relaxation results higher than 60% after just 30 minutes at 10 Hertz. A further 30 patients had sessions in theta (5 Hertz) and experienced relaxation states of 50-100%, after just five minutes, and significantly improved pain relief. [Shealy N, Cox R. In: Pain reduction and relaxation with brain wave synchronization (photo-stimulation). Study performed by the Forest Institute of Professional Psychology, Springfield, Missouri, 1990, 9pp.]

So you can see that flickering lights at the right frequency can have a profound effect on pain. We can make it a stronger effect by adding binaural beats.

But we can do more than that. We can add white light. Let me explain two more additions to this modality first.

Multi-Media Sensory Stimulation

We can add dreamy, slow, relaxing music. That can help a person in any state of mind to rapidly decompress and feel calm. The binaural beats can still be heard incidentally and will create a response, even if apparently obscured by the sound of the music. At the subconscious level, our auditory acuity picks up every sound nuance and our physiology responds, even if we cannot separate out the binaural beats.

Then we can also introduce creative guided imagery, through the sound of the spoken word. Through clever and enticing descriptions we may create beautiful and calming mindscapes; we can ask the listener to picture certain images, and define thoughts which we would like them to visualize for themselves, while relaxed and peaceful.

In this way, it's possible to encourage a person to re-program their feelings about pain or how they react to disease in their body. It's been called "transformational guided imagery" and "creative visualization and relaxation."

But we can also give more direct and specific instructions, to guide the individual into over-riding unpleasant messages from the body. Pain or discomfort of all kinds can be changed in character, till it's no problem, at all!

Take the "white light" meditation…

White Light Meditation

It has been discovered that white light in the brain overrides all perceptions of pain. It is not possible to feel pain while white light fills your brain. But it has to be white light in the mind, not just light shone into the eyes. This brain light is special and very healing.

It's a healing white fire, a cold fire, that burns away hurts and pain and negative feelings. This is a skill you can learn and, soon after doing so, you will just be able to think only the words "white light" for pain to go away rapidly.

It sounds very simple; and so it is. You need to learn the technique of switching on white light in your brain. Voice-guided imagery may give you specific instructions. If not, while relaxed and entering a theta state, try your own meditation.

The simplest method of all is to imagine a ball of white light (you will be lying down). Place it "above" your head (just beyond the skull confines). For those of you in the know, this is the crown chakra, of course. Get the idea of the blazing white light burning up all pain and ills. Draw it down into your skull. Feel it burning away the pain.

Then let the ball of white light slowly descend through your body, burning away all hurts and inflammation; it's white fire but not hot, so it leaves the tissues cool and pain-free. Slowly push the light all the way down your body, through the pelvis, past the hips, down the thighs and legs, and into the feet.

Finally, slowly, push it out of the body altogether, beyond the tips of your toes, and let it go…

It may take some days, or even a few weeks, to fully master this ability. But it's worth the effort of learning it and you will begin recovering right away, as from NOW. Even slight results at visualizing white light will bring increasing degrees of release from pain, healing, and recovery.

Thought Transformation

Another powerful method of healing we can borrow from Tibetan Buddhism: it's called *thought transformation*. This method allows a person to see the problem or sickness as something positive rather than negative. A problem is only a problem if we label it a problem. If we look at a problem differently, we can see it as an opportunity to grow or to practice, and regard it as something positive. Even pain can be wrestled to the floor, using this kind of pragmatic psychology.

If someone gets angry at us, we can choose to be angry in return or we can choose to be thankful to them for giving us the chance to practice patience and tolerance! It takes a lot of practice to master these methods, but it can be done.

This can be important in how we relate to disease and pain. For example, if the doctor announces that we have cancer, or a slipped disc, or a broken leg, we tend to respond with the relevant mindset, complete with what we consider to be the appropriate symptoms, feelings and pains.

But it is possible to transform our perceptions and thereby to make the experience far less negative. Children are the model for this. Do you remember how each day held excitement and delight? You couldn't wait to get up and rush out to play. Every day was a new adventure. The world was filled with possibilities and tomorrow was not important; just the moment you were in was important.

Sometimes you got bruised or hurt but it never seemed to last; do you remember that?

See, children feel very little pain; their minds are not tuned to real pain. Oh, they hurt, of course. They cry and wail a little. But then something distracts them and they soon forget the pain. Their minds quickly become engrossed in something else instead; whatever it is that interests them.

There were tears, real tears, but then suddenly there are smiles and laughter, as if nothing had happened.

But—here's the point: the body didn't heal that fast; the bruise or graze or sprain didn't suddenly vanish. The injury is still there. But the child doesn't feel it. Though the body hasn't changed, the mind has!

That's what alpha and theta states are about.

The Hardware

There are a number of devices on the market that are capable of creating brain entrainment through binaural beats, photic driving, music, and creative voice imagery.

My favorite at this time is the Kasina, from Robert Austin's Mind Place. *Kasina* is a Sanskrit (actually *Pali*) word which refers to an ancient system of meditation that uses visual objects to focus the mind.

The Kasina has perfect build quality and its presentation (unboxing as the Americans say) is very attractive.

A built-in an MP3 player and an 8-GB microSD card are included, with over 50 audiovisual excursions, with aural backgrounds ranging from the soothing sounds of nature to ambient electronic tapestries to embedded binaural beats and isochronic pulses, all beautifully orchestrat-

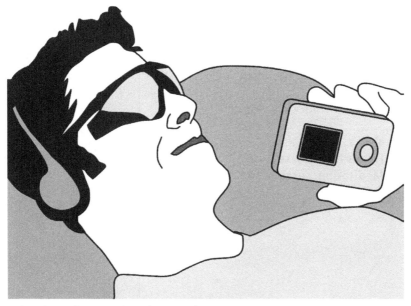

ed and synchronized to the visual experience.

You can also listen to tracks by me, particularly a white light meditation, which you should find helpful for mastering any kind of pain.

The Kasina also features a backlit, colored LCD display, a built-in rechargeable lithium battery, and can be used as a USB external audio device. It's also the most capable AudioStrobe decoder on the market, with 16 different color-mapping presets. Use the Color Organ feature to turn any music into a colorful light show - and it includes six different settings, to help match the mood of your music. And the GanzFrames (glasses) feature six colored LEDs per eye, for an even more intense experience, should you desire.

What I like especially is that you are not tied to tracks only from the Mind Place website. You can load any mp3 of your own choosing. You can put your playlists up there! The Kasina includes a free editor app for both Mac and Windows, on the included flash memory card.

Imagine a world of pure, jewel-like color illuminating your visual and mental fields. Amazing visual effects can be produced, including the illusion of complex, shifting geometrical patterns. This imagery, in combination with soothing, flowing sounds, can be so compelling that the mind clears of extraneous thoughts. In this way, the Kasina experience is a form of meditation.

Pain? What pain?

You can order a Kasina unit from my website, with a $25 discount ($325 plus shipping). Just enter the code: PAINGUIDE.

www.alternative-doctor.com/pain

See also:
- **Hypnotherapy, section 15.**
- **Meditation, section 24.**

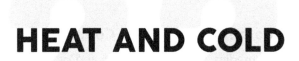

HEAT AND COLD

It's a little-known fact among doctors and physiologists—and even neurologists—that pain is a mixture of hot and cold sensation. You can produce very distinct pain by combining the two sensations in the skin.

All the more surprising, therefore, that both heat and cold seem to offer a partial solution to pain. Warmth is comforting for may pain sufferers. But be aware that for others, warmth makes the pain worse and they seek a cooling sensation.

Heat helps soothe stiff joints and relax muscles. Cold helps numb sharp pain and reduce inflammation. You can use temperature therapy to complement meds and other healing modalities in this text. It's simple to do, affordable, soothing -- and you have to sit down to use either one, so add relaxation.

Packs and Compresses

For short-term pain relief, you can make a pack from items such as:

- An electric heating pad
- A gel pack that can be microwaved or frozen
- A bag of ice or frozen vegetables

Whether trying hot or cold relief, wrap the pack in a towel to help protect your skin. Even ice packs can "burn" your skin and produce unpleasant discoloration.

Or make a compress -- a washcloth or small towel soaked in hot or cold water, wrung out, and folded. Cover with a dry towel to insulate it.

Apply to the painful area for 15-20 minutes several times daily.

Soothing Heat and Ice Compounds

A number of remedies, such as menthol and/or salicylate topical sprays, sticks, foam, liniments. and ointments, are designed to simulate the feeling of heat and/or cold. Salicylate, particularly, gives a warm spreading sensation, rather like burning but just short of discomfort. Menthol, on the other hand, is associated with coolness. Camphor is sometimes added.

Salicylic acid (aspirin), from the white willow, I have already discussed in section 2. Topical applications, such as oil of wintergreen, are the methyl form.

Menthol is obtained from cornmint, peppermint, or other mint oils. It has local anesthetic qualities, and it is widely used in pastilles to relieve minor throat irritation.

Camphor comes from the wood of the camphor tree (*Cinnamomum camphora*), a large evergreen tree found in Asia (particularly in Sumatra, Borneo and Taiwan), which is related to cinnamon. Camphor (in "Vick's") has a topical soothing effect but also works by inhalation of the vapors.

Menthol, camphor and methyl salicylate work by increasing blood flow and they are known as *counterirritants*. They work by causing the skin to feel cool and then warm. These feelings on the skin distract you from feeling the aches/pains deeper in your muscles, joints, and tendons.

Hence names like "Deep Heat" (30% methyl salicylate & 8% menthol), "Tiger Balm" (camphor 11%, menthol 8%), and "Icy-Hot Patches," menthol 5%.

This approach can be used for temporary relief of minor aches and pains of muscles and joints, such as sprains, bruises, backache, and arthritis.

Use topically ONLY. These soothing substances are nevertheless toxic when swallowed.

If you are using the lotion, spray, or foam, shake the bottle well before using.

Don't overuse remedies of this kind; if the pain persists, try to find some other method of relief. There is more than a suspicion that rub-on and rub-in liniments, ointments, and sprays may release enzymes that can further damage joints.

Apply a thin layer of medication to the affected area no more than 3 to 4 times a day. Rub in gently and thoroughly. After applying the medication, wash your hands unless you are using this medication to treat the hands. If treating the hands, wait at least 30 minutes after applying the medication to wash your hands.

It is important not to apply these substances, especially camphor, to broken or irritated skin (e.g., cut, scraped, sunburned), because it can enter the body quickly and reach concentrations that are high enough to cause poisoning.

Also, be aware that heat can increase the risk of side effects. Do not apply these medications immediately before, during, or after activities that increase skin temperature (e.g., bathing in hot water, swimming, sun bathing, heavy exercise) or in hot/humid weather. Wait until your skin has cooled before applying the medication. Do not use a sunlamp/tanning bed, hot water bottle, or heating pad on the treated area.

Allergic reactions are rare. However, seek immediate medical attention if you notice any symptoms of a serious allergic reaction, including rash, itching/swelling (especially of the face/tongue/throat), severe dizziness, or trouble breathing.

Capsaicin

Finally, if you want really hot, you can consider Mexican chili!

Capsaicin is the chemical found in chili peppers that gives them their hot, spicy taste. It's also the active ingredient in several over-the-counter pain products, including Capzasin HP, Sloan's Liniment, and Zostrix. The burning sensation from capsaicin is supposed to do more than just get your mind off the pain, although it does that quite well.

In theory, neurons shut down after they've been stimulated by the chemical (The Gate-Control Theory, page 5), so the burning and other unrelated sensations—including pain—cease. In fact the results from studies testing the low concentrations of capsaicin present in most OTC products (less than 0.1%) haven't been impressive.

One problem is that people don't like the chili burning sensation, so they don't stick with the treatment. Moreover, capsaicin is poorly absorbed, so the low concentrations don't deliver enough of the chemical to neurons to dependably produce the desensitization that is supposed to make capsaicin more than a distracting irritant.

High-dose capsaicin patches have been developed, but they require local or regional anesthesia. In other words, stronger preparations CAUSE pain. That makes them wholly inappropriate for the treatment of chronic pain.

The bottom line: the over-the-counter capsaicin products may not be effective for many people.

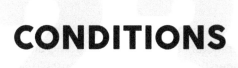

CONDITIONS

Back Pain

They say that back pain is the number one reason people around the world go to the doctor. If that's the case, it seems strange that there is so little that orthodox medicine can do. However, I have lot of good, workable—and you'll see very novel ideas—about treating back pain or backache. You'll find something here that will work for you, I'm sure.

Let me start with a dire warning: never, EVER allow surgery on your back. No laminectomies, no fusions, no touch, leave-well-alone. The results are so bad, so uniformly unhelpful, and even damaging, that you will wish you never had. There is even an official name for messed up back surgery, it's called "failed back surgery syndrome" (FBSS), which refers to chronic back and/or leg pain that occurs after back (spinal) surgery. No matter the many arguments assembled by the surgeons who want your money; they are all false. They may try to paint a nice pretty picture. But do not allow yourself to be suckered into the trap. Say NO! It's not safe and it's rarely, if ever, successful and, once it goes wrong, Mother Nature cannot help you with a fix.

You'd be better to just go on slugging yourself with knockout painkillers than going in for surgery. But there are really quite a number of things you can consider.

CHIROPRACTORS AND OSTEOPATHS

You've heard of the people who will "manipulate" backs, I'm sure. Maybe you are wondering if they are good? After all, osteopaths and chiropractors were fought tooth and nail by doctors, for more than a century; that must mean they are charlatans, surely?

Not a sound argument. Doctors just want to protect their turf and get any competition out of the way. Eventually in 1987, chiropractors in the US won a massive battle against the AMA, and successfully established that doctors were in an unlawful conspiracy in restraint of trade.

But, just as there are good and bad doctors, there are bad (and some very bad) chiropractors and osteopaths. Some are just wizards and, with a deep understanding of the body's musculo-skeletal dynamics, can just do a quick twist-click-shove and all of a sudden a patient who walked in crippled with pain can stretch comfortably and walk out minus all discomfort.

Unfortunately, they are not all as good as that. My wife Vivien had some back trouble a few years ago. She went to see a local chiropractor in northern Nevada, who was supposed to be very good—he wrote books and taught classes to other chiropractors. Sadly, he was incompetent. My wife was not helped; his techniques didn't work; his stupid advice to keep ice packs against her spine for hour after hour produced actual skin damage; but there was no real relief.

We finally had to get Vivien on a plane to London (family matters) and while she was there she managed to get an appointment with another chiropractor, a woman who clearly knew what she was doing. That practitioner instantly spotted something important that the American "expert" chiropractor had missed and fixed Vivien's problem (a misaligned pelvis) at once. My wife has had no further trouble.

That's about the spectrum that you can expect to encounter.

I urge you to be specially wary of those practitioners who use a spring-loaded metal punch device, that they use to bang around on the spine with. It's not just bad, it's dangerous. Your spine is so delicately balanced in dynamics that even just stroking it in the wrong way can put it out of balance. So the idea of doing the equivalent of banging along your backbone with a metal hammer in the pretense of doing some good is not just absurd, it's criminal.

These stupid devices (called an "activator") costs $750, so of course the chiropractor wants to get value out of it. Just run for the door if you see one.

In fact if the practitioner, whether chiropractic or osteopath, doesn't have fingers as smooth as silk while touching your spine, run for the door!

I mean it!

VARIETIES OF BACK

Back pain is a big topic; it ranges from sciatica (pain down the back of the leg but originating in the spine), to a stiff and painful neck. In between, there's scoliosis (bent spine), herniated ("slipped") disc, and sacroiliac joint problems. The key concept in all of these conditions and other symptoms of backache lies in spasm.

When a spinal nerve is squeezed or trapped, it leads to a protective muscle spasm. The body is trying to hold the backbone still, so that further painful squeezing or crushing of the nerve doesn't happen. Unfortunately, after a very short time, the spasm itself becomes painful.

Surprisingly (and you won't read this in many places!), the original hurt may have gone; the only thing keeping the back pain going is the spasm itself. How do I know? Because countless times I have switched off the back pain completely in just minutes by relieving the spasm and—presto!—the pain was already gone.

How Is This Done?

Let me start with the long, involved method that got me started. I painted the back with iodine (Lugol's iodine is fine). Almost immediately, it is possible to see that one spinal segment, like a band round the body, is pale and discolored from the rest. That tells you at exactly what level, what vertebra, the problem lies.

I then got the patient to carefully and painlessly adjust their spine and posture until they felt comfortable. There is always one sweet spot, where the pain passes off. Lo and behold! At that moment the colored band (caused by unequal sweating) disappeared, too.

I then had the patient hold that position as long as possible; up to fifteen minutes, if he or she could keep still long enough. In that time the spasm passed off, because there was no need for the protective mechanism. Once the spasm was gone, so was the pain. The wary patient stands up and finds to their immense relief that the pains have disappeared.

It's important to realize the severity of the pain is not related to the severity of tissue damage; it's related to the intensity of the spasm, that's all.

YOU CAN DO THIS

OK, here's a version of this technique you can do yourself, at home, without bothering with the iodine dye marker.

Just lie flat on the hard floor (no cushions, no bed, nothing soft, though a blanket is OK to lie on, if you don't have carpet).

Lie on your back, with arms by your side, spread a little outwards from the body, palms upwards. We call this the anatomical position. OK, that will probably hurt but be careful; take your time. Once you are in position, then you go to work, trying to find that magic sweet spot, where the pain disappears. There is always such a position; trust me, just be patient and find it.

Don't make any large of violent movements; you might hurt yourself. Just gently and slowly wriggle, trying different positions for your hands, spine and legs. When you get to the sweet spot, enjoy! Just lie there as long as you can. If you stay pain free for 15 - 20 minutes, you'll probably find you can get up (with help if necessary).

There may be a little residual soreness but if you are extremely careful and respectful of your body's signals, and do nothing to trigger the sharp pain for a few hours, you'll find that life will start to get back to normal.

INVERTERS

You've just learned the secret of why inverters often help. By hooking your feet in the stirrups and hanging head downwards, you are in effect stretching your spine. To do so reduces any pressure on nerves, which is good, but it also draws on the muscles, which eventually let go due to fatigue, thus relaxing the spasm.

It's that simple.

Yes, inverters work. But if you can master the technique of finding your sweet spot, you don't need to go in for the expense of an inverter. It's up to you.

MAGNESIUM INJECTIONS

I have to mention this one! There was a time when I thought most of my clinical ecology colleagues were giving each other IV magnesium shots for back pain. I wasn't into it, because I didn't have any problem. But a number of colleagues did.

It can be IM but better by far is 1 gram (1,000 mg) of magnesium sulfate, injected slowly into a vein. It's quite safe but there is a curious warmth sensation, which starts at the back of the throat and spreads. Don't be alarmed, it passes off in less than a minute.

There are no side effects but you need to stay sitting for a few minutes afterwards, because it drops your blood pressure significantly. For some people that mean a transient dizziness. Better to be patient than faint!

Don't just keep repeating the treatment. Get to work on finding and eliminating your inflammatory foods (section 32).

OTHER THERAPIES

Many of the other therapies for pain featured in this book at perfectly sound and can be tried. These include neural therapy, biopuncture, massage, aromatherapy, and SCENAR.

Headache and Migraine

A migraine is a very bad headache that tends to recur. With a migraine, you may feel nauseated and might vomit. The pain is usually on one side of your head (hemi-crain in French) and you may be very sensitive to bright lights and noises. Moving around can make the headache feel worse. There are many forms of migraine headaches. Classic and common are the two major varieties.

Headache and even migraines can be caused by temporomandibular joint (TMJ) problems; chiropractors will say they are due to cervical subluxations and the like; but what I learned in the early 1980s is that over 90% of headaches and migraines are caused by inflammatory food reactions.

Some things can trigger a migraine or make it worse. Headache triggers can be things you eat, smell, hear, or see.

Stress and time pressure, major hassles, major losses, anger, and conflict are also possible triggers. We sometimes called them "tension headaches."

But one type of migraine is especially worthy of mention: abdominal migraine. It directly connects gut and cranium. It's gonna be food!

Classic food triggers include the five "Cs": chocolate, caffeine, claret (any red wine), cheese, and citrus (orange, etc.) I would add a sixth "C" trigger, which is commoner than all the other five put together: cow's milk.

One of my outstanding cases was a lady of 63 years, who had had migraine all her life (60 plus years). It turned out to be cow's milk… and *only* cow's milk. Was she grateful for the discovery? No, she was mad as hell. All those wasted days of her life and no doctor had ever even suggested it might be something she was eating!

MORE PARTICULARS

Migraine is often preceded by an "aura." The aura is the occurrence of neurological symptoms 10-30 minutes before the classic migraine attack. Effects you may see are flashing lights or zigzag lines or you may temporarily lose vision. Other symptoms of migraine can include speech difficulty, confusion, weakness of an arm or leg, and tingling of face or hands.

The pain of a classic migraine headache is described as an intense throbbing or pounding felt in the forehead/temple, ear/jaw or around the eyes. Classic migraine starts on one side of the head, but may eventually spread to the other side. It's usually very severe (enough to interrupt normal living) and an attack may last one to three days.

Typically, a patient will want to withdraw and lie down in a darkened, quiet room.

Painkillers have variable and often little impact. Prescribed drugs include ergot-related compounds and Tegretol. Now there are newer, more effective drugs available - Imitrex, Zomig, and Maxalt are some choices for relief of the pain of migraine. For headaches that occur three or more times a month, preventive treatment is often recommended. Drugs used to prevent classic and common migraines are available by prescription.

Herbal remedies include feverfew (page 113), which is famously good for migraine, but better at prevention than cure.

Conventional thinkers are obsessed with faulty models, which only partly explain the problem and do not give rise to a total cure.

Doctors think migraines may be caused by a chemical or electrical problem in certain parts of the brain. A key element of a migraine headache is blood flow change in the brain. According to theory, the nervous system responds to a trigger such as stress by creating spasms in the nerve-rich arteries at the base of the brain. The spasms constrict several arteries supplying blood to the brain, including arteries from the scalp and neck. As these arteries constrict, the flow of blood to the brain is reduced. At the same time, platelets clump together and release a chemical called serotonin. Serotonin acts as a powerful constrictor of arteries further reducing blood and oxygen supply to the brain. In reaction to the reduced oxygen supply, certain arteries within the brain dilate to meet the brain's energy needs.

Doctors believe this dilation causes the pain of migraine. "Migraine headaches tend to run in families, suggesting that genetic factors contribute to a person's susceptibility to migraines." (UpToDate, 2006).

The problem is, it doesn't lead to really valuable therapy. It's a theory, rather than a treatment!

FOOD ALLERGY
There is no question in my mind that food allergy or hypersensitivity is the number one cause of migraine. You must strive to identify and eliminate the culprit foods. Section 32 tells you how to do this.

After teaching this for many years, I was gratified when a team of doctors, under professor John Soothill at the Great Ormond Street Hospital in London, UK, published a paper explaining a trial in which they had proved that 93% of migraine was food allergy. [Egger J, Soothill JF, Carter CM, et al. Is migraine food allergy? A double-blind placebo-controlled trial of oligoantigenic diet treatment. *Lancet*. 1983; 2: 865-869.]

Incredibly, fools argued with me "that was only children" and denied that the facts applied to adults. It was like saying a scientific trial only applied to the people involved! Anyway, within a short space of time, confirmation arrived that it applied to adults too. [Carter CM, Egger J, Soothill JF. Food allergy and adult migraine: Double-blind and mediator confirmation of an allergic etiology. *Ann Allergy*. 1985; 55:126-129.]

TRIGGERS
Even foods are just triggers, though the most rewarding to deal with since, as soon as the person gives up eating the foods, the migraines or headaches tend to vanish.

Of course the classic "5 C's" and dairy are not the only possible food allergens. Others include:

- Aged cheese
- Bananas, figs and raisins
- Beer, wine, and hard liquor
- Fermented and pickled foods such as pickled herring
- Monosodium glutamate (MSG), which is found in Chinese food, Accent seasoning, Lawry's Seasoned Salt, canned soups, TV dinners, processed meats, and some processed nuts and snack chips
- Nuts and peanuts
- Onions
- Pea pods or pods of lima beans
- Processed meats, deli sandwich meats, hot dogs, and other nitrite-containing meats
- Saccharin or aspartame in diet foods or diet sodas and drinks
- Sulfites in shrimp and processed potatoes, like boxed mashed potato mix
- Yeast-containing products, such as fresh breads and donuts

There are other triggers you could search for:

- Smells and fumes, tobacco smoke, light glare or dazzle, weather changes.
- Monthly periods, birth control pills, estrogen therapy; too much, too little, or interrupted sleep
- Excessive activity

MEDICINES THAT MIGHT TRIGGER A MIGRAINE
Certain medicines may cause migraine. Talk to your provider before you stop taking a medication.

- Cimetidine (brand name: Tagamet)
- Estrogens (including birth control pills)
- Fenfluramine (brand name: Pondimin)
- Indomethacin (brand name: Indocin)
- Nifedipine (brand name: Adalat, Procardia)
- Nitroglycerin (brand name: Nitrostat)
- Pain medicines in general (either overuse or withdrawal from them)
- Reserpine-containing medicines
- Theophylline

TREATMENTS OTHER THAN AVOIDANCE OF TRIGGERS
It has always seemed best to me to avoid any known triggers. Why court trouble? But some practitioners like to take a different route and train the patient to "cope" in other ways:

Women are very susceptible to migraines (about three times more commonly than men). Sometimes the problem doesn't come on till puberty. It may be made worse by pregnancy or even relieved by pregnancy. That suggests to some practitioners to work on hormone balancing and the monthly cycle.

Other approaches include:
- Biofeedback training
- Stress reduction
- Regular exercise, such as swimming or vigorous walking

Temporary relief can sometimes be obtained by using cold packs or by pressing on bulging arteries found in front of the ear or the painful side of the head.

Beware of help groups and websites, which are usually fronts for drug companies and their products.

Arthritis (All Types)

The word "arthritis" means inflamed joints and it can come in many forms, including osteoarthritis, rheumatoid arthritis, gout, and auto-immune disease, such as lupus.

Let's face it, the benchmark for aging is often perceived to be arthritis. As we get older, it seems inevitable that we get a little stiffer, which eventually turns to pain when we move. Finally our joints deform and we adopt the characteristic posture of an older, hunched person, perhaps needing a walking cane or frame.

It doesn't have to be like that, because so many people reach 90 and beyond without crippling arthritis. In fact some nonegenarians and centenarians are remarkably supple and move quite freely, so pain is not inevitable.

Not all forms of arthritis are connected with aging. The dreaded rheumatoid arthritis, for instance, is an autoimmune disease that can strike at any age. In this type of inflammation, the body seems to be attacking itself, like an allergy to dust, feathers, or pollen, but antibodies are made against the body's own joint tissue. The result is inflammation, pain, and incapacity. Autoimmune diseases seem to be reaching epidemic proportions and some people feel that our toxic environment and unhealthy lifestyles may be to blame.

I am among those physicians who even suspect that this may be due to modern very intense vaccinations programs, damaging and confusing the immune system early on, so that it never quite functions as it should but is busy reacting inappropriately, to food and environmental triggers.

However, the more familiar type of osteoarthritis that attacks older people is regarded as mainly due to wear and tear. It attacks different joints on the whole. The inflammatory arthritis tends to attack the fingers and can cause a great deal of damage, even deformity, such that the sufferer has difficulty gripping or even holding objects, without marked pain. Osteoarthritis on the other hand creates joints surrounded by crusty bone extensions but does not much deform the line of movement.

It's not the purpose of this section to describe all the many variants of arthritis. But if you are unlucky and it has struck, at any age, you might like to consider the possible options. The low inflammatory foods diet, for example, is one of the few healing modalities that is found to produce remarkable recoveries in the rheumatoid pattern of arthritis conditions.

That's not surprising, since avoiding inflammatory foods will settle down inflammation and inflammation is the cause of joint pains and the generalized feeling of malaise that goes with this type of arthritis.

That said, all these remedies can be applied to any arthritic condition, with an expectation of some benefit and pain relief. Let's look through them; all are described in this book.

PHYSICAL CONTACT THERAPIES

Massage and aromatherapy are soothing and tend to reduce the perception of pain. Don't allow any practitioner to take the "physiotherapist's approach," which is to pull, twist and force movement, in spite of the pain which exists to prevent further joint damage.

More is not better in this context.

Osteopaths and chiropractors are a far safer bet.

DEVICES

You can try electronic devices, such as the SCENAR or a TENS machine. I have often told the story of the very first time I ever used a SCENAR.

I had just bought one, the instructions were all in Russian and I barely knew how to switch it on!

Undaunted, I visited a friendly patient, an elderly lady, whom I had successfully helped with her asthma, using the food allergy elimination approach. This was in Spain. She had a twinge of arthritis in both knees but simply put it down to age and it never worried her or limited her activities.

"Let's try an experiment," I suggested. "I'll treat only your left knee with this new device, tomorrow we can compare that with the right knee and see how well it worked." She agreed, so we duly did a 15-minute treatment on her left knee, using only the basic settings.

Next morning, when I dropped by, she told me delightedly the pains had gone from BOTH knees. Moreover, both knees stayed pain-free until I left Spain and returned to England, some three months later.

HERBAL REMEDIES

You may have heard of herbs for arthritis. Some are very famous. The main ones that come to mind are:

Aloe Vera. Aloe is one of Nature's most healing plants. Try it for burns, especially sunburn. You will learn right away that aloe reduced inflammation! That's what we want for arthritis. Also, incidentally, aloe contains glucosamine, which is a natural compound found in cartilage. Glucosamine is a known treatment for arthritis pain and stiffness.

Boswellia (Indian frankincense). Gum resin is used, from the bark of the Boswellia tree found in India. It reduces inflammation and treats rheumatoid arthritis (RA), osteoarthritis (OA), and bursitis symptoms. In a 2004 study, people who took Boswellia reported less knee pain, better mobility, and an ability to walk longer distances than those taking placebo. A 2008 British review found Boswellia safe and effective for both osteoarthritis and rheumatoid arthritis.

Cat's Claw. Cat's claw is a plant, not an animal product! There are two species: *Uncaria tomentosa* is most commonly used in the US and *Uncaria guianensis* is typically used in Europe. Medicine is made from the root and bark. Both species are effective for improving symptoms of both osteoarthritis and rheumatoid arthritis (WebMD). Do not confuse cat's claw with cat's *foot*.

Turmeric (*Curcuma longa*): Turmeric is an extremely effective anti-inflammatory herb and thus an effective pain reliever. It contains at least two chemicals (curcumin and curcuminoids) that decrease inflammation (and are very much like the oft-prescribed non-steroidal anti-inflammatory drugs, or NSAIDs).

Licorice (*Glycyrrhiza glabra*): Licorice acts much like your body's own natural corticosteroids (which reduce inflammation). Licorice decreases free radicals at the site of inflammation and inhibits the enzyme production that's involved in the inflammatory process. Reducing inflammation definitely helps arthritis.

Nettles (*Urtica dioica*): Surprisingly, despite their stinging property, nettles are very nutrient-dense (you may have heard of nettle soup). They can contribute to strong bones while easing the pain of arthritis. While NSAIDs may sometimes seem a necessary evil for arthritis, using nettles may help you reduce the dose to a safer level.

HOMOTOXICOLOGY
You can read about homeopathy and complex homeopathy (homotoxicology) in section 8.

One arthritis remedy that stands out, however, is Zeel from the company HEEL (Traumeel can be pretty good too).

Rather than just rely on this one remedy, it's better to engage with a skilled practitioner and work on overall recovery of health, using detox, drainage, and maybe even miasms.

Don't forget also biopuncture therapy, which is built on homotoxicology remedies (section 8). It can be very effective for pain of all kinds, not just arthritis.

DON'T FORGET THE REST
Finally, you must face the fact that losing weight and taking regular exercise is a MUST. The body is dynamic and plastic; it responds to use. Heck, you can even grow new brain cells by thinking hard! You can surely repair your joints somewhat by putting them to use. Just don't play squash or racket ball, OK? *Excessive exercise actually increases inflammation.*

In fact, keeping moving is essential for the inflammatory-type arthritis, otherwise you seize up. But even the wear-and-tear arthritis is benefitted by some movement. Think of an old car crock: it's better to keep driving it around, however slowly, than to leave it parked up and motionless. You know that.

In fact a recent study was able to show that knee arthritis, for instance, was benefitted by around 6,000 steps per day. We do approximately 100 steps per minute, so that equates to roughly an hour of walking. But that's not just exercize; it means all walking. So movement around your home, to and from the car, etc. counts towards the total.

An easy way to count steps is to buy a pedometer, which records all the steps you make. You can also get a cell phone app that does the same thing.

The study, published June 12, 2014, in Arthritis Care & Research, tracked the number of steps taken over a week by adults who were at risk for knee arthritis or already had it. All used pedometers and were part of a large osteoarthritis study.

Two years later the researchers assessed any arthritis-related functional limitations. They found that for every 1,000 steps taken, functional limitations were reduced 16 percent to 18 percent.

The point is that the less one moves, the weaker the muscles get, and the less stable the joints are, increasing inflammation and pain. Sitting around also increases the risk of weight gain, which can adversely affect joints.

In the end, the foods you eat will prove to be the single biggest factor in the symptoms you experience. It's very rare that it doesn't produce a dramatic improvement in joint health. See, joints are extremely sensitive to toxins. The tiniest trace of anything deposited between the two silky smooth-gliding ends of the bones will produce marked pain. That includes deposits of antigen-antibody complexes, which I described on page 210.

Once you have identified and eliminated your bandit foods, be sure to eat plenty of fresh, raw foods, especially brightly colored foods rich with antioxidants, to protect your body from the effects of free radical damage, which is a significant factor in aging.

HEALTHY FATS AND OILS
Omega-3 oils are particularly important for arthritis, especially fish oils EPA and DHA. Vegetable sources, such as alpha-linolenic acid (ALA) from flax and borage, have conversion challenges. Due to minor ge-

netic variations encountered in some countries, ALA can progress to EPA easily but conversion of ALA to DHA may only be minimal. This puts DHA as a number one dietary requirement: if you can't make it, you have to swallow it.

What this is about is that omega-3 fatty acids make helpful and soothing prostaglandin series 1 (PGE-1). Omega-6 fatty acids, on the other hand, convert to prostaglandin series 2 (PGE-2), which causes pain and inflammation. Unfortunately, omega-6 fatty acids heavily predominate in the typical diet. Junk found is loaded with it. But beware: farmed tilapia and other fish species can contain more omega-6s than a cream doughnut!

Generally speaking, foods that are not organic and naturally grown have major nutritional liabilities of this sort. Eat as close to nature as you can and only whole food (not been processed).

Omega-3 fatty acids have many other health benefits, but reducing inflammation is vital to pain sufferers.

AUTOGENIC TRAINING AND MEDITATION

I put these two together because autogenic training has been very suitably described as a Western meditation technique. The idea is that both are very powerful ways of controlling the mind and what the mind allows itself to register as pain.

Remember, all pain is central in the end. Pain is not peripheral, in the firing of the pain nerve fibers from the tissues, but how the brain and mind interpret those firings.

Does it work? You bet. You only have to consider those pictures you must have seen of Eastern fakirs sticking skewers into their tissues or eating razor blades to realize that the mind has formidable powers of interpreting experience in any way it chooses.

The Western mystics who used physical pain to remind themselves of their holy commitment are a similar example. Christians have been notorious for hair shirts, self-flagellation, starvation, asceticism, and even being crucified on a modern-day cross. It borders on sadomasochism but one thing is clear: if you want it to happen to you, pain can be made to seem something desirable.

Theologians try to explain that the redemptive value of pain makes it lovable in its effects, even though pain by itself is not. Pain is temporal and limited, thus to undergo it is worthwhile to gain the real benefits. For those with this viewpoint, pain is seen as a means to an end. Thus, a modern Catholic saint, Josemaria Escriva, founder of Opus-Dei, said while consoling a dying woman who was suffering in a hospital, "Blessed be pain! Glorified be pain! Sanctified be pain!"

To the rest of us, it's a bit weird. I only make the point that you can alter your experience of pain very profoundly by how you think about it.

Meditation

There is an embarrassment of choices in what type of meditation to adopt. You make your own choice, basically. I cannot honestly report that some are better than others. It's horses for courses. Being comfortable and enjoying what you do will prove far more beneficial than trying to practice a technique which does not sit well with you, just because it's supposed to be "better."

Buddhist Vipassana meditation is hugely popular in the West. It's all about "being present," letting your mind run, and accepting whatever thoughts come up, while practicing detachment from each thought. Mindfulness is taught along with an awareness on the breath, though the breathing is often considered to be just one sensation among many others, not a particular focus.

Transcendental Meditation™ is more proprietary and you may have to swallow gobbets of Maharishi-worship to get accepted in its circle of followers. It has been extensively studied, however; you can find details of its valued properties in *The Physiology of Consciousness* by Robert Keith Wallace (a joint publication of the Institute of Science, Technology and Public Policy and Maharishi International University Press, Iowa, USA, 1986).

As neuroscientists have studied meditation, they've discovered some interesting ways in which it affects the physical structure of the brain. These include effects that can be seen in autonomic functions and neurotransmitters as well as changes in blood flow and brain wave activity.

A 2011 paper published in the *Journal of Neuroscience* (Apr 6, 2011) suggested that the effects of meditation on pain, after only an hour of training, could be even more powerful than morphine!

According to the lead researcher, Fadel Zeidan, PhD, post-doctoral research fellow at Wake Forest Baptist Medical Center, meditation can dramatically reduce both the experience of pain and pain-related brain activation. There was a big effect: about a 40% reduction in pain intensity and a 57% reduction in pain unpleasantness.

"Meditation produced a greater reduction in pain than even morphine or other pain-relieving drugs, which typically reduce pain ratings by about 25%," said Zeidan.

For the study, 15 healthy volunteers who had never meditated attended four 20-minute classes to learn a meditation technique known as *focused attention*. Focused attention is a form of so-called mindfulness meditation, where people are taught to attend to the breath and let go of distracting thoughts and emotions.

Both before and after meditation training, brain activity of the study participants was examined using a special type of brain scan. During these scans, a pain-inducing heat device was placed on the participants' right legs. This device heated a small area of their skin to 120° Fahrenheit, a temperature that most people find painful, over a five-minute period.

The scans taken after meditation training showed that every participant's pain ratings were reduced, with decreases ranging from 11 to 93 percent.

At the same time, meditation significantly reduced brain activity in the primary somatosensory cortex, an area that is crucially involved in creating the feeling of where and how intense a painful stimulus is. The scans taken before meditation training showed that activity in this area was very high. However, when participants were meditating during the scans, activity in this important pain-processing region could not be detected.

The research also showed that meditation increased brain activity in areas of the brain known to shape how the brain builds an experience of pain from nerve signals that are coming in from the body.

It seemed that the more these areas were activated by meditation, the more that pain was reduced. Evidently meditation seems to work in various pain-processing parts of the brain, not just one, and that may be the key to its effectiveness. [Zeidan F, Martucci KT, Kraft RA, Gordon NS, McHaffie JG, Coghill RC. Brain mechanisms supporting the modulation of pain by mindfulness meditation. *The Journal of Neuroscience.* 2011; 31(14): 5540-5548.]

What's remarkable about this study is that it showed that very little training produced such an enormous benefit. Something to try, for sure.

Autogenic Training

Autogenic training is a mind control technique for autosuggestion and deep relaxation, developed by the German psychiatrist Johannes

Heinrich Schultz (1884-1970) and first published in 1932. During each session, the practitioner will repeat a set of visualizations that induce a state of relaxation. Each session can be practiced in a position chosen from among a set of recommended postures (for example, lying down, sitting meditation, slumped in a comfortable chair). The technique can be used to alleviate many stress-induced psychosomatic disorders and calm the response to pain.

Herbert Benson, MD, a Harvard professor also did significant research into this approach. He called it the "Relaxation Response" and wrote an influential book with that same title.

Autogenic training has been subject to clinical evaluation from its early days in Germany and from the early 1980s worldwide. In 2002, a meta-analysis of 60 studies was published in *Applied Psychophysiology and Biofeedback*, finding significant positive effects of treatment when compared to controls over a number of diagnoses; finding these effects to be similar to best recommended rival therapies; and finding positive additional effects by patients, such as their perceived quality of life.

Autogenic training was popularized in North America, particularly among practitioners, by Wolfgang Luthe, who co-authored, with Schultz, a multi-volume tome on autogenic training. Luthe was a firm believer that autogenic training was a powerful approach that should only be offered to patients by qualified professionals.

However, I consider it perfectly safe for self-taught therapy.

Like many similar techniques (progressive relaxation, yoga, qigong, varieties of meditation), autogenic training takes time to learn. But some biofeedback practitioners shortened the process by taking the most basic elements of autogenic imagery and developing "condensed" simplified versions that could be used in combination with biofeedback devices.

This was done at the Menninger foundation by Elmer Green, Steve Fahrio, Patricia Norris, Joe Sargent, Dale Walters, and others; they took the hand-warming imagery of autogenic training and used it as an aid to develop thermal biofeedback (warm extremities are an indication of deep relaxation).

There is no question about its capability to modulate the response to pain. The only issue would be the length of time it takes to truly master it.

I found a paper on PubMed from a midwives' journal that proposed the widespread application of autogenic training for some of the more common pain-allied disorders, such as childbirth, headaches and migraines, back pain, cancer and palliative care, and cardiology. Autogenic training was also able to reduce substantially drugs dependency.

A paper in the *Journal of Psychosomatic Research* declared autogenic training effective for tension headaches and comparable to hypnotism.

How It Works

It is not appropriate to try and give you a comprehensive guide to the training in a book of this nature, but here is an outline guide.

Basically, autogenic training is a series of auto-suggestion commands (hence the name). The would-be participant lies down on a sofa or bed or sits comfortably in a slouching chair.

With eyes closed and feeling relaxed, he or she then recites along these lines, repeating each phrase several times, until it begins to take effect:

1. My left arm is heavy. My right arm is heavy. Both of my arms are heavy.
2. My right leg is heavy. My left leg is heavy. Both of my legs are heavy.
3. My body feels heavy. My body is sinking into the bed. My body feels like lead.
4. I feel warm. My arms are warm. My legs are warm. My arms and legs are warm.
5. My heartbeat is slow and regular.
6. My breathing is calm, relaxed and regular.
7. My forehead is cool.

From this point on, the abilities shift to cognitive postulates and get more difficult. You should consult a text for further details.

But already you can add pleasant imagery and positive word suggestions for pain control.

I can report that I use this technique successfully myself, for deep relaxation, and you can soon train your body to respond to the instructions. I have even produced a CD to help get you started:

http://www.informed-wellness.com/free_cd/

I certainly think it's easier for us Westerners than trying to "wipe away thoughts" and "keep an empty mind," or other tricky conceptual auto-suggestions, as in meditation.

See also Hypnotherapy, section 15.

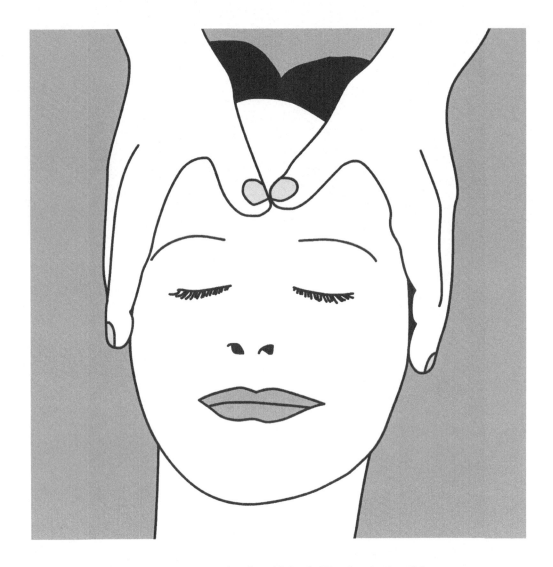

It surprises most people to be told the skull is quite plastic and de-
forms from pressure. Nevertheless, it's true. This is the key to cra-
nio-sacral therapy: the practitioner puts pressure on skull bones,
in certain directions, and these pressures are directed within.

It's healing capability has been demonstrated many times over,
even if we can only partially explain how it works.

Plus CS therapy feels wonderful!

CRANIOSACRAL THERAPY

CranioSacral Therapy is an exceptionally gentle yet extremely powerful form of treatment, increasingly recognized for the depth of its influence, and the comprehensive range of its therapeutic effects.

The main characteristic of CranioSacral Therapy is the correction of micro-movements of the cranial bones through micro-manipulation. With that manipulation the therapist can influence other structures, all the organs and systems of the body.

CranioSacral Therapy primarily facilitates processes that enhance the body's innate abilities for natural healing. The main goal is to improve the flow of cerebrospinal fluid. Improving fluid motion and exchange specifically enhances the functions of the brain; spinal cord; autonomic control systems; visual, auditory, olfactory and gustatory sensory systems; motor and motor co-ordination systems; endocrine system; and the immune system. Less directly, it seems to affect all other body systems; therefore, it is exceptionally useful for most chronic conditions and as a preventive measure.

CranioSacral Therapy has been shown to alleviate a wide range of conditions, including:

- Headache, migraine, insomnia
- Chronic neck pain, back pain, persistent pain anywhere in the body
- Asthma, bronchitis, sinusitis
- Tinnitus and middle ear problems, ENT problems
- Chronic fatigue, lack of energy
- Stress, tension, anxiety, emotional and depression related difficulties
- Hormonal imbalances

- Cardiovascular disease, high blood-pressure, vertigo

- Motor coordination impairments

- Orthopedic problems

- Dental and Temporo-Mandibular Joint (TMJ) problems

- Traumatic brain and spinal cord injuries

- Post Viral Fatigue Syndrome (PVFS), myalgic encephalomyelitis (ME), glandular fever

- Post-surgical dysfunction

plus all kinds of digestive, mental, behavioral and learning problems.

The Anatomical Basis Of Craniosacral Therapy

The medical basis of CranioSacral Therapy is a recently discovered physiological system, the craniosacral system that can be found in all living being with brain and spinal cord, and it begins functioning in the womb and continues its function until death. The name "craniosacral" is derived from the system's associated bones. Included are those of the cranium (skull, face and mouth) and of the spinal column which extends down to the sacrum, the triangular bone between the hips.

The system meets the criteria of classification as semi-closed and hydraulic. It contained within a tough waterproof membrane, called Dura Mater, which surrounds and protects the brain and the spinal cord. In the head this dural membrane attaches to all the cranial bones; in the spine attaches to the 2nd and 3rd bones of the neck, the sacrum and coccyx (tailbone).

An important function of craniosacral system is the production, circulation and reabsorption of cerebrospinal fluid (liquor) that maintains the physiological environment in which the brain and nervous system develop, live and function. All the nerves in the body originate somewhere along the pathway of the dural membrane system. Restrictions - occurring from physical or emotional events - along this pathway may impede the flow of the cerebrospinal fluid, thereby causing pain at some point in the body.

All the bones attached to the dural membrane move constantly as the cerebrospinal fluid is pumped in and our; each bone has its own course of movement. When a particular bone moves off course or does not move at all, that indicates that there is a restriction in the flow of the cerebrospinal fluid. An imbalance in this system can adversely affect the development of the brain and spinal cord, which can result in sensory, motor and neurological dysfunction.

The craniosacral system works in conjunction with other body systems such as the cardiovascular, respiratory, musculoskeletal, endocrine and nervous system. There is no part of the body that is not affected by the functioning of the craniosacral system.

The Craniosacral Rhythm

The craniosacral system, like the cardiovascular and respiratory systems, has its own palpable rhythm, called the craniosacral rhythm or craniosacral pulse. The normal craniosacral rate is 6-12 cycles per minute, which remains unaffected by emotions, exercise and so on. The motion of the cranial bones is transferred to and taken up by the peripheral bones of the body, the connective tissue and all the organs. Hence, the motion becomes a whole body motion. The motion of the cerebrospinal fluid creates a pulse that called the craniosacral rhythm.

A trained craniosacral therapist can palpate this rhythm to evaluate the movement of the cerebrospinal fluid throughout the body as well as to detect any variances or possible restrictions in the flow of the cerebrospinal fluid. When a restriction has been found, the therapist will assist the natural movement of the fluid and related soft tissue to help the body self-correct, to develop spinal flexibility and to improve general health and well-being.

Summary

CranioSacral Therapy is completely different from standard massage and structural forms of chiropractic and osteopathic adjustments. The movements, used during the session, are extremely subtle, sensitive and gentle; they are not at all sharp, hard or quick. The therapist follows the body's natural waves and rhythms to effect a change in the body.

CranioSacral Therapy is a subtle and profound healing form, which encourages the body's natural mechanisms to improve the functioning of the brain and spinal cord, dissipate the negative effects of stress, and enhances general health and resistance to disease.

WHAT IS ROLFING®
STRUCTURAL
INTEGRATION?

Rolfing is named after its creator, Ida Rolf (1896- 1979), a biochemist from New York City who studied alternative methods of bodywork and healing beginning in the 1920s.

Rolf began developing her system in the 1920s to help the chronically disabled who had been unable to find help elsewhere. Her main goal was of organizing the human bodily structure in relation to gravity. This method was originally called "Postural Release" and later "Structural Integration", also commonly known as "Rolfing".

Dr. Rolf developed a theory that the body's aches and pains arose from basic imbalances in posture and alignment, which were created and reinforced over time by gravity and learned responses among muscles and fascia — the sheath-like connective tissue that surrounds and binds muscles together. Rolfing developed as a way to "restructure" muscles and fascia.

Because chronic stress often leads to tension in the upper back, neck and shoulders, Rolfing can help the body break these patterns that contribute to chronic discomfort.

The focus on manipulating fascia is part of what distinguishes it from chiropractics, which deals largely with bones, and from therapeutic massage, which works on muscles.

Essentially, the Rolfing process enables the body to regain the natural integrity of its form, thus enhancing postural efficiency and your freedom of movement.

What are the benefits?

Rolfing Structural Integration has the ability to dramatically alter a person's posture and structure. Rolfing can potentially resolve discomfort, release tension and alleviate pain. Rolfing aims to restore flexibility, revitalize your energy and leave you feeling more comfortable in your body. The genius of the work rests on Dr. Rolf's insight that the body is more at ease and functions most effectively when its structure is balanced in gravity.

Athletes, dancers, children, business professionals, and people from all walks of life have benefited from Rolfing. People seek Rolfing as a way to ease pain and chronic stress, and improve performance in their professional and daily activities. It's estimated that more than 1 million people have received Rolfing work.

Research has demonstrated that Rolfing creates a more efficient use of the muscles, allows the body to conserve energy, and creates more economical and refined patterns of movement. Research also shows that Rolfing significantly reduces chronic stress and changes in the body structure. For example, a study showed that Rolfing SI significantly reduced the spinal curvature of subjects with lordosis (sway back); it also showed that Rolfing enhances neurological functioning.

Studies have shown that those with neurological impairments such as carpal tunnel syndrome, piriformis syndrome and pronator syndrome can benefit from this structural realignment. Rolfing may be able to relax tissues contributing to jaw pain in the temporomandibular joint or TMJ.

The term "Rolfing" is now a registered service mark in 38 countries.

How It Works

The most commonly known system of Rolfing is called the "Ten Series," which is broken up into three different steps. The first three sessions, known as as "sleeve" sessions, focus on loosening and rebalancing surface layers of connective tissue. Breathing techniques are suggested to enhance the quality of breath during the session.

Bodywork is typically first done on arms, chest and the abdominal wall, specifically focusing on the diaphragm. It then includes the back and neck as well as moving downward toward the upper legs and buttocks.

The second and third sessions finish out the legs and focus on how the body - in context with the head, shoulders and hips - relates to itself in space.

The next four sessions, known as the "core" sessions, focus on the body from the head down to the pelvis and the deep tissue of the legs.

The final three sessions are known as the "integration" step, in which the goal is to achieve balance, movement and coordination within the entire network of the body. Sessions are typically scheduled weekly, but can vary depending on the client and therapeutic goals.

Often there is a short discussion following the treatment to determine outcomes and suggest a home program.

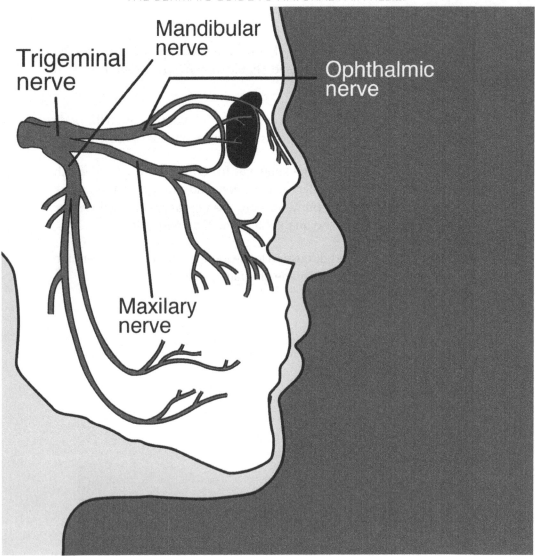

The trigeminal nerve is a sensory nerve covering the face and side of the head. It has many smaller branches, such as the lingual nerve and branches to the eye orbit and sinuses. When your head hurts due to sinusitis, or toothache, that's the trigeminal nerve.

This important nerve serves the teeth and gums, via the maxillary and mandibular branches. So when the trigeminal is irritated, anywhere along its many pathways, the pain which results can travel widely and appear far from the actual source of irritation. Remarkably, an abscess under a tooth in the lower jaw can feel as if it is in the upper jaw or even the forehead! This spreading effect of pain is called "referral".

[The muscle movements of the head and face are caused by a different nerve: the facial nerve, which is the one that gets hit with botox therapy]

TRIGEMINAL NEURALGIA (TIC DOULOUREUX)

Trigeminal neuralgia is a chronic pain condition that affects the trigeminal nerve, which collects sensations from the head and face. It is a severe pain, usually affecting only one side of the face at a time. It is generally held that the trigeminal nerve "imagines" the pain (so-called neuropathic pain) and that it does not relate to any structure served by the nerve.

This is far from true. Oftentimes, the real cause is a hidden dental lesion. More of that in a moment. First: The condition and its orthodox treatment.

The typical or "classic" form of the disorder (called "Type 1" or TN1) causes extreme, sporadic, sudden burning or shock-like facial pain that lasts anywhere from a few seconds to as long as two minutes per episode. These attacks can occur in quick succession, in volleys lasting as long as two hours.

The "atypical" form of the disorder (called "Type 2" or TN2), is characterized by constant aching, burning, stabbing pain of somewhat lower intensity than Type 1. Both forms of pain may occur in the same person, sometimes at the same time. The intensity of pain can be physically and mentally incapacitating.

The trigeminal nerve has three branches, serving:

- the upper head and face
- the cheeks, nose and maxilla (upper jaw) and
- the lower jaw, teeth and gums, and bottom lip.

Both sides of the head can be affected by the disorder but this is not usual.

Causes

TN is associated with a variety of conditions, such a blood vessel pressing on the trigeminal nerve as it exits the brain stem. This compression causes the wearing away or damage to the protective coating around the nerve (the myelin sheath). TN symptoms can also occur in people with multiple sclerosis, a disease that causes deterioration of the trigeminal nerve's myelin sheath.

Rarely, symptoms of TN may be caused by nerve compression from a tumor, or a tangle of arteries and veins called an *arteriovenous malformation*. Injury to the trigeminal nerve (perhaps the result of sinus surgery, oral surgery, stroke, or facial trauma) may also produce neuropathic facial pain.

The common causes are rarely even considered (see below).

Quality of Pain

People who suffer this condition are well aware of the extreme savagery of the pain at times. It can be like having a knife stabbed into the face or jaw (and then twisted some!)

The quality may range from sudden, severe, and stabbing to a more constant, aching, burning sensation. The intense flashes of pain can be triggered by vibration or contact with the cheek (such as when shaving, washing the face, or applying makeup), brushing teeth, eating, drinking, talking, or being exposed to the wind.

The pain may affect a small area of the face or may spread. Bouts of pain rarely occur at night, when the affected individual is sleeping.

Attacks may stop for a period of time and then return; the condition can be progressive. The disorder is not fatal, but can be truly debilitating. Due to the intensity of the pain, some individuals may avoid daily activities or social contacts because they fear an impending attack.

It's commoner in people over age 50, although it can occur at any age, including infancy.

Treatment

Anticonvulsant medicines—used to block nerve firing—are said to be effective in treating TN1 but often less effective for TN2. These drugs include carbamazepine, oxcarbazepine, topiramate, gabapentin, pregabalin, clonazepam, phenytoin, lamotrigine, and valproic acid.

Tricyclic antidepressants such as amitriptyline or nortriptyline are often resorted to deal with the pain.

Eventually, if medication fails to relieve pain or produces intolerable side effects such as cognitive disturbances, memory loss, excess fatigue, bone marrow suppression, or allergy, then surgical treatment may be recommended.

DO NOT ALLOW SURGERY without exploring the important origins of this condition that I am about to describe.

TMJ and Dental Focus

The hidden triggers of this condition that are missed, time and time again, lie with the teeth and jaw bones. Even if the pain is felt elsewhere, do not be fooled. Pain often radiates, meaning it spreads out from its origins. It can be very difficult to detect where exactly the pain is originating. The stabbing pangs can be coming from the teeth, yet felt in the temples. It is important to have a knowledgeable practitioner to help, who understands to search widely for hidden causes.

First of all, make sure it's not some other conditions that get missed: post-herpetic neuralgia (nerve pain following an outbreak of shingles), cluster headaches, and temporomandibular joint disorder (TMJ, which causes pain and dysfunction in the jaw joint and muscles that control jaw movement).

Because of overlapping symptoms and the large number of conditions that can cause facial pain, obtaining a correct diagnosis is difficult, but finding a cause of the pain is important as the treatments for different types of pain may differ.

So, after they've done a scan to make sure you don't have a tumor or arteriovenous anomaly, *get a good holistic dentist to search for NICO.*

NICO: What's In A Name?

It stands for Non-Ischemic Cavitational Osteonecrosis. Wikipedia gives it as Neuralgia-Inducing Cavitational Osteonecrosis but in my pioneer days, back in the 1980s, we used the former name and I'm sticking with that. Here's what the 1996 Research and Scientific Affairs Committee of the American Association of Endodontists had to say about it:

The NICO lesion (Neuralgia-Inducing Cavitational Osteonecrosis, also known as Ratner's bone cavity) was first described in the dental literature in 1920 by G.V. Black. The lesion consists of ischemic osteonecrosis found in the jaws of patients with symptoms of atypical facial pain or trigeminal neuralgia. Research has shown the lesions to be difficult to diagnose. The lesion will sometimes present very subtle radiographic changes often detectable only by a technetium scan or with multiple periapical radiographs. The overlying soft tissues show no changes. Many etiologies for NICO have been suggested, but none have been substantiated through research. According to noted oral pathologist Dr. J.E. Bouquot, the typical NICO case occurs as facial pain many years after an extraction or an infection in the area… The recommended treatment for NICO is decortication and curettage of the bony tissues. While this practice has produced relief of pain in some cases, NICO has a strong tendency to recur and to develop in other jawbone sites. Most affected sites with a postoperative NICO diagnosis have been in edentulous areas. However, some patients with long, frustrating histories of pain associated with endodontically treated teeth have been presented the treatment option of tooth extraction followed by periapical curettage in an attempt to alleviate pain. The American Association of Endodontists cannot condone this practice when NICO is suspected. Because of the lack of clear etiological data, a NICO diagnosis should be considered only as a last resort when all possible local odontogenic causes for facial pain have been eliminated… if possible, periradicular surgery and curettage should be attempted, not extraction.[AAE Position Statement on NICO lesions (Neuralgia-Inducing Cavitational Osteonecrosis)". AAE Research and Scientific Affairs Committee. Retrieved 8 May 2013]

It is accurate to say this position paper is now out of date. The "correct" or best-practice treatment would be curettage, followed by effectively sterilizing the cavity, using free oxygen or ozone, and perhaps using homeopathics to encourage natural healing.

Low level infra-red or laser light therapy (see section 14) can also be used successfully.

Bone grafts are rarely necessary; Nature herself is pretty good at recovery and restoration.

NICO can cause atypical facial neuralgia, trigeminal neuralgia, chronic sinusitis, phantom toothache pain, and headaches including migraines plus widespread adverse health effects. It needs to be tracked down with any of these pain conditions.

Research by Dr. Boyd Haley (former Chairman, Department of Chemistry, University of Kentucky) show that ALL cavitation tissue samples he's tested contain toxins, which significantly inhibit one or more of the five basic body enzyme systems necessary in the production of energy (Toxins Produced by Oral Microorganisms and Their Toxic Effects on Critical Enzymes in the Human Body, ALT, http://www.altcorp.com/AffinityLaboratory/bacteriatox.htm).

These toxins, which are most commonly likely to be metabolic waste products of anaerobic bacteria (bacteria which don't live in oxygen), may produce significant systemic effects, as well as play an important role in localized disease processes, which negatively affect the blood supply in the jawbone.

Other Dental

Endodontic cysts are also commonly occurring usually in the gums at the tip of a tooth, that have pockets of bacterial infection that can cause inflammation and pain in some cases similar to cavitations. Bacterial infections are also known to have systemic effects.

According to Stuart A. Geene DDS, the most misunderstood area in all of endodontic surgery is the notion that all cysts must be completely removed to promote healing. If root canal problem is completed, then the cystic area will reverse. Therefore, 100% enucleation of the cyst is not necessary. If the cyst starts to encroach on sensitive anatomy, only a portion of it should be carefully removed. A cystic area will not recur following complete sealing of the apex.

If a cyst is removed, it should be sent it for a biopsy (if it's worth taking out, it's worth sending out for biopsy). This is standard of care in the endodontic community.

Cracked or otherwise damaged teeth can also result in severe pain. Often the tooth has been opened for drainage, but there is no relief.

The tooth remains exquisitely painful to the touch. Sometimes there is accumulated pus which, as soon as it is released, leads to immediate comfort.

The take-home message is: for pain anywhere in the head and jaw area, seek the help of a competent biological dentists, not a card-carrying dental mechanic. You can find such individuals via the International Academy of Oral Medicine and Toxicology (www.IAOMT.com)

You can also learn more from DAMS, the dental amalgam and mercury study group:

http://www.flcv.com/dams.html

REFLEX SYMPATHETIC DYSTROPHY SYNDROME (RSDS)

Reflex sympathetic dystrophy syndrome, also known as complex regional pain syndrome, is an uncommon disorder of the sympathetic nervous system that is characterized by chronic, severe pain.

The so-called sympathetic nervous system is that part of the autonomic nervous system that regulates involuntary functions of the body such as increasing heart rate, constricting blood vessels, and increasing blood pressure. Excessive or abnormal responses of portions of the sympathetic nervous system are thought to be responsible for the pain associated with reflex sympathetic dystrophy syndrome.

Its counterpart is the parasympathetic system, also part of the autonomic nervous system. The two (sympathetic and parasympathetic) have largely polarized functions and balance each other out.

The symptoms of reflex sympathetic dystrophy syndrome can be very severe but typically begin mildly, with burning pain, especially in an arm, fingers, palms of the hands and/or shoulders.

In some individuals, RSDS may occur in one or both legs or it may be localized to one knee or hip. Frequently, this condition is be misdiagnosed as a painful nerve injury. The skin over the affected area may become swollen (edema) and inflamed. Affected skin may be extremely sensitive to touch and to hot or cold temperatures, a condition called cutaneous hypersensitivity.

The exact cause is not fully understood, although it may be associated with injury to the nerves, trauma, surgery, atherosclerotic cardiovascular disease, infection, or radiation therapy. Its inflammatory nature is the key to resolving it.

THE ULTIMATE GUIDE TO NATURAL PAIN RELIEF

Treatment

Start always with removing inflammatory foods. Often, a simple appraisal of the diet, with elimination and challenge testing (page 220), leads to an immediate breakthrough.

Also, nutritional anti-inflammatories, like omega-3s can work wonders. Correct any out point noted.

As for specific therapies, Dr. Frank Shallenberger MD recommends Prolozone®, a proprietary therapy, which he developed. It is a variant of prolotherapy (Section 30).

The basis is a homeopathic/oxygen-ozone treatment, excellent for all forms of musculo-skeletal and joint pain including chronic neck and back pain, rotator cuff injuries, degenerative and arthritic hips and knees, degenerated discs, and shoulder and elbow pain.

Part of the protocol is a connective tissue injection therapy of collagen producing substances and ozone gas, which can reconstruct damaged or weakened connective tissue in and around joints.

Prolozone® causes repair and tightening of the lax structures, partially torn connective tissue and ligaments. It also reduces the pain/inflammation cycle. This allows for better circulation, increased blood flow carrying nutrition, and hydration of the damaged tissues, leading eventually to an increased range of motion and decreased pain.

The result could be a lasting cure, because in many cases Prolozone® actually corrects the underlying pathology of the disorder, and it is claimed to be up to 75% successful.

David Steenblock, a US osteopath, has other suggestions. He says the first treatment to try is a combination injection of 1 ml of adenosine, 1 ml of methylcobalamine (10,000 micrograms/ml) and 1 ml of Nexavir (if you can afford it).

Dr. Jacob Teitelbaum reports seeing 'dramatic improvement' with regular use of the drug but notes that regular treatment can be difficult given its expense ($500 per month). He also notes that symptoms may return after the drug is discontinued. Dr. Lapp calls it a 'wonderful alternative' with the proviso that its expensive and the shots can be painful.

If can't get the Nexavir (formerly known as kudapressin) then just go with 1 ml of B-complex and 1-3 ml of procaine if needed to blunt the pain of the injection. This is given daily and in severe cases can be given every 12 hours. Steenblock states this should work in most cases within 1-2 days.

Next to try would be DMSO: Section 29.

All other pain therapies are possibilities to try.

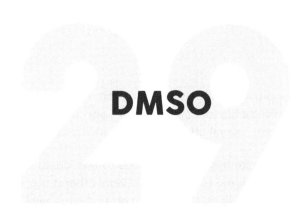

DMSO

DMSO, or dimethyl sulfoxide, is a by-product of paper making. It comes from a substance found in wood. It has been used as an industrial solvent since the mid-1800s. From about the mid-20th century, researchers have explored its use as an anti-inflammatory agent.

This surprise use dates from the 1960s, when Stanley Jacob, MD, head of the organ transplant program at Oregon Health Sciences University in Portland, was investigating compounds that might help preserve organs for transplant. DMSO attracted his attention because of the way it penetrates skin without damaging it. He experimented with DMSO and found that it could relieve pain.

From the start, DMSO was highly controversial—and some were worried that this "miracle" drug had harmful side effects, although nothing specific was found. By the mid-1960s, DMSO was a popular product in health-food stores. It was inexpensive—and it worked!

DMSO is a prescription medicine and dietary supplement. It can be taken by mouth, applied to the skin (used topically), or injected into the veins (used intravenously or by IV).

According to WebMD, DMSO can be used to decrease pain and speed the healing of wounds, burns, and muscle and skeletal injuries. DMSO is also used topically to treat painful conditions such as headache, inflammation, osteoarthritis, rheumatoid arthritis, and severe facial pain called tic douloureux.

It is used topically for eye conditions including cataracts, glaucoma, and problems with the retina; for foot conditions including bunions, calluses, and fungus on toenails; and for skin conditions including keloid scars and scleroderma.

It is sometimes used topically to treat skin and tissue damage caused by chemotherapy when it leaks from the IV that is used to deliver it. DMSO is used either alone or in combination with a drug called idoxuridine to treat pain associated with shingles (herpes zoster infection).

The FDA has approved DMSO as a prescription medication for treating symptoms of painful bladder syndrome. It's also used under medical supervision to treat several other conditions, including shingles.

It is very safe, despite hysterical reactions to one death by the FDA, an Irish case, in which the patient took several other drugs. The actual cause of death was never established. No other deaths have even been attributed to DMSO. Taken properly, it's safer than the vast majority of pharmaceuticals.

However, it has one unpleasant side effect: it stinks. When you use it, you will stink too!

Mode Of Action

DMSO is recognized as a potent anti-inflammatory in its own right and that can help relieve many kinds of joint or muscle pain, such as strains, and joint and muscle aches.

Why is it so effective? First, DMSO has analgesic properties and reduces pain quickly—which is why it is great for rubbing on sore muscles and joints. Laboratory studies suggest that it decreases pain by blocking peripheral nerve C fibers.

Also, DMSO reduces inflammation by acting as an antioxidant—and so it neutralizes some of the free radicals that promote inflammation. Some evidence suggests that it also can ease swelling, further helping with aches and pains.

Finally, DMSO is rich in sulfur, one of the most abundant elements in your body, playing a major role in the formation collagen, the most vital chemical component of connective tissue—the tissue that joins and supports all our body tissues. Collagen also makes up cartilage. Lack of sulfur has been shown to be a factor in cartilage deterioration and several arthritic conditions.

You will already know, maybe without knowing, that sulfur is very healthful! It's the principle beneficial mineral in spa waters. Health-seekers from around the world flock to the rejuvenating waters of natural sulfur springs. The warm, mineral-rich waters relieve chronic pain and inflammation, facilitate healing, and improve function and range of motion. Since most of us don't have our own sulfur hot springs nearby,

DMSO treatment is a great alternative for restoring sulfur levels and relieving pain.

DMSO creams are available from health-food stores and online. To use, simply rub a small amount into the affected area until absorbed. Use 70% strength, to avoid skin irritation.

Your practitioner, if he or she is familiar with DMSO, may choose to inject it IV or provide you with a topical preparation.

PROLOTHERAPY

Similar in name to Prolozone (page 194) but different entirely in action is prolotherapy.

Prolotherapy, formerly known as sclerotherapy, is a treatment technique used for chronic myofascial pain, back pain, osteoarthritis, or sports injury.

Prolotherapy is the repeated injection of any substance that promotes growth of normal cells, tissues, or organs. Possible reagents include dextrose solution or other irritating substances into the joint, tendon, or painful tissue in order to provoke a regenerative tissue response. Similar techniques have been used for about a century, but the first formal publication describing prolotherapy dates back to 1956, by Dr. George Hackett.

According to Hackett, within the attachment of weakened ligaments and tendons to bone, the sensory nerves become so overstimulated by abnormal tension as to become not only the origin of specific local pain, but also referred pain throughout the body, possibly as far as the head, fingers and toes, from specific relaxed ligaments and tendons.

In other words, something like trigger points (page 45), which cause pain remote from their site and lightning reactions in neural therapy, which also cause distant pain. Hackett's belief was that support connective tissue has become weakned and needs strengthening. Causing scar tissue would, in a limited sense, lead to extra support (scar tissue is tough).

Therefore prolotherapy is designed to permanently strengthen the "weld" of disabled ligaments and tendons to bone by stimulating the production of new bone and fibrous tissue cells has been developed.

The original belief was that the injections formed scar tissue to stabilize the joint, tendon, or ligament. Nowadays, it as argued that the injections provoke the proliferation of tissue, allowing for limited regeneration.

The exact response to the injections is not currently known, and so explanations of mechanism remain speculative. This is not enough to condemn the treatment — something is physically happening and it is possible that a useful local phenomenon is occurring.

We don't know.

3 Types

We can identify 3 types of prolotherapy:

1. Injection of a known growth factor (a complex protein) that specifically begins growth of a certain cell line. This approach is in early stages of study for arthritis (growing cartilage cells) and sprain and strain (growing fibroblasts). It will likely remain a more expensive option than the next two approaches.

2. Injection of something that causes the body to produce its own growth factors. Non inflammatory (10% or less) dextrose is the most widely used. Two double blind studies have now shown that simple 10% dextrose injection is effective in arthritis. Growth factors produced include platelet-derived growth factor (PDGF), transforming growth factor-beta (TGFB), epidermal growth factor (EGF), basic fibroblast growth factor (bFGF), and connective tissue growth factor (CTGF).

3. Injection of something extra that causes activation of the inflammatory cascade to produce growth factors. These solutions often include dextrose plus phenol-containing-solutions and/or sodium-morrhuate-containing solutions.

The only double blind studies done thus far were small in scale and published in enthusiastic alternative health journals; not that convincing. I found one from *The Lancet*. In this study the control group received injection with multiple bone contacts which itself will stimulate growth factor release.

Another study, published in the journal *Rheumatology*, failed to show any real benefit but the technique was questionable.

Practitioners who use prolotherapy swear by it (but then, they would, wouldn't they?) Some patients are happy with it but then, as I have often said, patient testimonials are not science and do not free a therapy from the placebo problem.

It has been almost 60 years since Hackett's first edition describing pro-lotherapy. In that time prolotherapy has remained marginalized, with-out sufficient high-quality clinical research to clearly establish its effec-tiveness. One has to ask why is there so little clinical research, over such a long period of time?

Either researchers have been unable to obtain positive results with rig-orous trials, or those using prolotherapy are insufficiently interested in testing whether or not the treatment actually works.

So you try it on faith. The ultimate scientific test is: if it works for you, it works! (just kidding, but tread carefully)

References:

1. Reeves, K.D., and K. Hassanein. Randomized prospective dou-ble-blind placebo-controlled study of dextrose prolotherapy for knee osteoarthritis with or without ACL laxity. Alt Ther Hlth Med, 2000; 6(2): 37- 46

2. Reeves, K.D. and K. Hassanein. Randomized prospective placebo con-trolled double blind study of dextrose prolotherapy for osteoarthritic thumbs and finger (DIP, PIP and Trapeziometacarpal) joints: Evidence of clinical efficacy. Jnl Alt Compl Med, 2000; 6(4): 311-320

3. Ongley, M.J., et al. A new approach to the treatment of chronic low back pain. Lancet, 1987; 2: 143 - 146.

4. Dechow, E., et al. A randomized, double blind, placebo-controlled tri-al of sclerosing injections in patients with chronic low back pain. Rheu-matology, 1999; 38:1255- 9.

ANTI-INFLAMMATORY SUPPLEMENTS

Most chronic pain conditions have a strong element of inflammation in their make up.

In fact, anti-inflammatory medicines such as aspirin, ibuprofen, and naproxen work well because they block the enzymes that trigger both swelling and pain.

However, there are many natural food substances and supplements which also reduce swelling and inflammation, in some cases even better than NSAIDs.

According to G. Cole, UCLA Professor of Medicine and Neurology, reported to Newsweek Magazine in a Special Summer Issue in 2005 (pages 26-28):

"While anti-inflammatory drugs usually block a single target molecule and reduce its activity dramatically, natural anti-inflammatories gently tweak a broader range of inflammatory compounds. You'll get greater safety and efficacy reducing five inflammatory mediators by 30 percent than by reducing one by 100 percent."

Essential Fatty Acids

Gamma-linolenic acid (GLA) is an omega-6 fatty acid that is found mostly in plant based oils such as borrage seed oil, evening primrose oil, and black currant seed oil. Omega-6 fatty acids are considered essential fatty acids. They are "essential" for human health, because our bodies can't make them -- you have to get them through food.

Gamma linolenic acid (GLA) has fairly good science to show its helpfulness against inflammation.

But beware: there are several different types of omega-6 fatty acids. Most omega-6 fatty acids in the diet come from vegetable oils in the form of linoleic acid (LA). The body converts linoleic acid to GLA and then to arachidonic acid (AA).

Linoleic acid and arachidonic acid (AA) tend to be unhealthy because they promote inflammation. GLA, on the other hand, may actually reduce inflammation.

GLA taken as a supplement needs to be converted to a substance called DGLA that fights inflammation. Having enough of certain nutrients in the body (including magnesium, zinc, and vitamins C, B3, and B6) helps promote the conversion of GLA to DGLA.

Dose: see omega-3 recommendations below.

OMEGA-3S

Top of the line for fighting inflammation, without doubt, are the omega-3 series of essential fatty acids. The best sources are marine oils (fish oils, krill oil, etc.) and grass-fed beef. Yes, despite what you have read, eating beef can lower inflammation, if it's healthy beef and not from concentrated animal feeding operations (factory farms).

The main omega-3 fatty acid EPA, and to some extent DHA, are probably the most powerful anti-inflammatory substances we have.

Unfortunately, the standard diet in the Western world, loaded with synthetic and manufactured, processed foods, is very high in omega-6s (farmed tilapia fish, for example, has more omega-6 fatty acids than a cream donut). Therefore I find it convenient to say supplement only omega-3s, until or unless your diet is very rich in natural raw foods and already containing several sources of omega-3 series.

Dose: 2 – 3 grams daily (4 - 6 capsules). You must work with your doctor if you take any kind of blood-thinning agent; because omega-3s also slow blood clotting.

And the good news is that you can increase the anti-inflammatory effect of EFAs by adding in other natural substances, such as plants and herbs…

Anti-inflammatory plants and herbs

These include turmeric, green tea, ginger, rosemary, cat's claw, devil's claw, and willow bark. Because they work in the same way as NSAIDs, these pain supplements do pose similar risks, such as bleeding and stomach upset. However, the side effects tend to be less severe.

Turmeric is my favorite. By using it patients are often able to stop pain medications, such as NSAIDs, completely.

Vitamin D

A number of studies have linked low levels of vitamin D with increased levels of chronic pain. One 2009 study looked at the vitamin D levels of people with chronic pain who were using opioid painkillers. Those who had a deficiency of vitamin D needed almost twice as high a dose of medication to control their pain.

Get your doctor to check your serum vitamin D levels. Generally, below 50 ng per ml. is considered non-optimal and below 30 ng per ml is real deficiency.

Correct what is found. Supplementing 2,000 – 4,000 units daily is about right. Remember, you get more vitamin D via the skin, from exposure to good sunshine levels.

S-Adenosyl Methionine (SAMe)

SAMe is found naturally in our foods, however not in sufficient quantity to be therapeutic. It acts by, among other things, blocking the release of histamine and other inflammatory agents. There's good evidence that SAMe offers natural pain relief to people with osteoarthritis. Some studies have found that it's about as effective as prescription painkillers like Celebrex (a Cox-II inhibitor). But it's expensive: $80-$120 a month.

It is sold under numerous brand names in a variety of countries, including India, Russia, the USA, Italy, and several countries of the European Union.

Bromelain

The enzyme bromelain (extracted from pineapple), appears to reduce inflammation and pain. Some studies have found it helpful in osteoarthritis and knee pain. There's some uncertainty about how well it gets absorbed in digestion, given that it could be neutralized by stomach acid. More research needs to be done.

Papain

Similarly, the enzyme papain, from pineapple, is also a great anti-inflammatory. One study from Russia, listed on PubMed, significantly reduced the inflammation caused by a variety of test irritants, including: formaldehyde, dextrane and histamine. The researchers estimated that small doses of domestic papain (0.325 and 0.75 mg/kg) possess marked anti-inflammatory and hence analgesic activity to be at least equal to that of butadion (OTC) and indomethacin (Indocin).

Full On Enzyme Support

It is widely held in holistic medicine circles that taking a mixture of potent enzymes can dramatically reduce pain and inflammation. That's believed to be because it digests inflammatory substances in the blood and tissues. Makes sense, but nobody has ever proved that.

Good mixtures will include bromelain (from pineapple), papain (from papaya) and plenty of pancreatic enzymes, which include proteolytics (those which digest protein).

Wobenzym is an excellent formula, which I recommend a lot. It's quality but unfortunately that means it costs a lot. That's before you get into money conversions with the Deutschmark. You can take up to a dozen capsules per day. But don't just take more and more, without working at the reason why your system is loaded with inflammatory compounds.

Wobenzym, and similar formulas, work well on the pain of exercize recovery.

Astaxanthin

Astaxanthin is now regarded as the most powerful antioxidant found in nature. It comes solely from microalgae that produce it, and the sea creatures that consume the algae (such as salmon, shellfish, and krill).

Astaxanthin works better than beta-carotene, alpha-tocopherol, lycopene and lutein, all members of the same chemical family. It is a strong free radical scavenger and helps protect your cells, organs, and body tissues from oxidative damage and inflammation.

It is said to be over 500 times more potent than vitamin E at scavenging free radicals and 65 times more powerful than vitamin C.

Astaxanthin suppresses a variety of inflammatory mediators—including tumor necrosis factor alpha, a major prostaglandin and a major interleukin, nitric oxide, COX-1 and COX-2 enzymes. It takes longer to produce effects than NSAIDS, but this means it doesn't result in the dangerous side effects.

Despite its powers, there have been no adverse reactions among people taking astaxanthin.

Make sure your astaxanthin is the natural variety from marine algae—NOT the synthetic version. Real astaxanthin is more than 20 times more powerful as an antioxidant than the synthetic sort.

The recommend dose would be 8-10 mg per day. If you are on a krill oil supplement (which is rich in astaxanthin), you may need to take less on that account.

Whatever your pain condition, you might like to give astaxanthin a try. Or indeed any of the natural anti-inflammatories I have described here.

For more suggestions, see the section on Migraine (23).

THE NUMBER ONE CORRECTABLE CAUSE OF PAIN

If pressed to say what is the number one reason people experience pain in their bodies, I would surely have to point out the food allergy phenomenon or—these days—we would say inflammatory foods (sometimes I lapse into calling them "bandit foods"!)

We've already explained the connection between inflammation and pain. Add to that the fact that the commonest cause of inflammation is the food we eat and you'll see a pattern emerging…

Eating the wrong things will hurt you! The truth is I've "solved" the pain problems of tens of thousands of individuals—and lots more symptoms and conditions besides pain—by investigating foods that the person does not tolerate.

If you have headache, migraine, arthritis, bellyache (like irritable bowel syndrome of colitis), endometriosis, autoimmune diseases, and a whole host more of complaints, you need to work on the content of this section.

I'm not saying everything is *caused* by food intolerance but everything is *helped* by removing inflammatory foods. In many cases, that means a permanent cessation of the symptoms (at least provided you keep off the food).

If you have any kind of severe or intractable pain and no other effective solution has yet been found, you need to take this pathway.

Once-in-a-Lifetime Journey

Actually, I'm fond of saying everyone needs to make this journey at least once in a lifetime. For some, it's essential.

Every single individual human being needs to be familiar with this important health mechanism and how to keep it sweet to their own advantage. It affects us all to varying degrees but I'm record with the BBC as saying that everyone has at least one badly tolerated food; they just don't know about it.

See, everyone think foods are nice and safe and friendly; well, they nourish our bodies, don't they? How can something safe to eat be harmful?

Not so fast. Foods are a complex mixture of chemicals and many of these chemical substances are quite toxic, as we'll see in a moment. We have become adapted and able to eat these toxic foods only because of the discovery of fire. By cooking plants in particular, many hundreds of potentially poisonous foods become safe to eat.

But they may still be capable of setting up an inflammatory reaction. Take a look at some of the bad things in foods—and I'm talking about organic whole foods, not just junk from the supermarket.

Potato and tomato, for example, belong to the same family as belladonna, a deadly poison! Is that relevant? You bet; I have had patients in terrible pain due to both foods. One 40-something woman was so crippled with arthritis, she faced a lifetime in a wheelchair. But it was potato—and only potato—that caused her nightmare arthritis. Once she gave up eating it and switched to sweet potato (different botanical family) she was fine.

To learn to do this properly, you will probably need a more comprehensive guide, like my book **Diet Wise** (www.DietWiseBook.com) or even the video classroom version **Diet Wise Academy** (www.DietWiseAcademy.com)

But we can get started with your education right here and now. What follows are the basics:

Basic Inflammatory Mechanisms

Let me introduce you to just a dab of technical stuff, to help you better understand the connection between bandit foods and pain.

There are really four kinds of "allergy" reaction; actually we call it hypersensitivity, types I - IV. Let's use the proper terms.

Type I hypersensitivity is often the worst: it's sudden and sometimes severe. It's the sort of reaction that may put a person in hospital with dangerous anaphylaxis. Fortunately, it's rare and needn't bother us here.

But types II, III, and IV are much slower, subtler and lingering. It's more a build-up effect—and patients will often use that very expression.

Type III especially, is associated with what we call "immune complexes" circulating in the blood (antigen-antibody clumps). These settle in the tissues and can produce pain all through the body and a feeling of general unwellness (malaise). It's a condition similar to *serum sickness*. That's when you get a wrong blood transfusion and your body goes into overload and shock.

The answer is to transfuse only blood that has been specifically tested for safety against the patient's own type; "test and cross-match," as we doctors say when ordering it.

The similarity to food reactions is heightened when you learn that blood grouping is done with lectins and these substances occur through our foods but some are especially loaded with tricky lectins (see below).

Natural Toxins in Foodstuffs

To those who think "plants" are safe, natural, and nurturing, I like to point out that deadly nightshade (belladonna), opium, hemlock and digitalis are all herbs – but very dangerous indeed!

Nice tasty fruits contain liver-toxic fructose and all those pretty colors and delicious flavors in fruits come from what we call phenolic compounds, closely related to drain cleaner (phenol or carbolic acid). Green coffee bean, for example, contains chlorogenic acid; it may have beneficial properties, to do with controlling blood sugar, but some individuals are highly intolerant of it.

Several foods contain nicotine, which is not good for anybody (milk, banana, beef, cheese, chocolate, tomato, potato, and other foods in the nightshade family).

Other poisons include prussic acid (cyanide) and its precursor amygdalin, nicotine, solanin, atropine, oxalic acid (in rhubarb), cucurbitacins (in zucchini), and a host of others.

In fact, Nature has seen fit to endow a number of plants with the capacity to synthesize substances that are toxic to humans and other animals. Ingesting them may produce unpleasant consequences which are not allergic but may become confused with an allergy.

Farmers and veterinarians, who are more advanced in this health issue than most doctors, have known for years that animals become sick if they graze on certain types of plant (for example, bulls become enraged if they eat loco weed – "loco" being Spanish for crazy). Many plant substances are toxic to humans in quite small quantities, including deadly nightshade, acorns, and hemlock. Ricin, the toxic principle in caster seeds *(Ricinus communis)*, is one of the most poisonous substances known: a minute drop on a needle at the tip of an umbrella was used in an infamous political assassination on the streets of London in 1978.

The fact is that all plants, including edible ones, contain quantities of poisons. Carrots, for example, contain a nerve toxin: *caratotoxin.* And someone once pointed out that if cabbage had to undergo the tests that drugs are now subjected to before being pronounced fit for humans, it wouldn't pass. Obviously, most often the amounts of poison in foods are tolerable. Toxicity is a matter of degree.

Alkaloids

These are small organic molecules, usually comprising several carbon rings with side chains, one or more of the carbon atoms being replaced by nitrogen (which confers the alkalinity). About 7 to 10 per cent of all plants contain alkaloids, of which several thousand are now known.

Famous alkaloids include nicotine, quinine, strychnine, ergotamine, and atropine. The less toxic ones, such as caffeine, are used for pleasant social effects. The powerful ones are hallucinogens (cannabis, LSD and mescaline).

We have already talked about endorphins or the body's natural morphine-like substances (page 9). Certain foods contain alkaloids that are called *exorphins,* meaning morphine-like compounds from outside the body.

The well-known food allergy effect of addiction, where withdrawal from the food causes unpleasant symptoms, may be due at least in part to the addictive properties of exorphins present in the food.

The action of alkaloids on the nervous system is generally to disrupt electrochemical transmission at nerve junctions (synapses), either preventing transmission (as in the case of the plant poison *curare*) or enhancing it inappropriately (as, for example, physostigmine). Locoism, referred to above, is of this latter class.

Outbreaks of food poisoning due to solanine (from potatoes), tomatine (tomatoes), and dioscorine (yams) have all been reliably observed in either humans or domestic animals. Death due to alkaloid overdose is fortunately uncommon in humans; in Socrates' case (hemlock) it was deliberate murder by the state. But subclinical alkaloid intoxication occurs all the time. The 'edible' nightshades (potatoes, tomatoes, capsicums, and peppers) are especially rich sources, but cabbage, peppercorns, and many other foodstuffs are not far behind.

Exorphins

These are morphine-like peptides derived from partially digested grain, milk, and legume proteins. Pharmacologically they behave, when tested on isolated tissues, very much like morphine, hence the name. It is reasonable to propose that, in people whose intestinal digestion of these foodstuffs is incomplete, exorphins are absorbed and have the effect of a small dose of an opiate drug - for example, patients who take wheat bran and find that their constipation gets worse. On the plus side, the well-known effect of pleasant somnolence after a meal is probably also due to morphine-like activity.

Caffeine Family (Methylxanthines)

It is commonly forgotten that caffeine and theobromine (which occur in tea and coffee) are toxic substances. Taken in sufficient quantities, they can cause cerebral edema (so-called "water on the brain"), convulsions and even death, though no one has ever been able to establish that tissue damage can be caused by chronic ingestion at normal levels.

Methyl xanthines are a notorious cause of headache and, if that is your problem, you will need to investigate that possibility in the pages that follow.

These substances can also cause a painful cystic breast condition called chronic cystic mastitis or fibroadenosis (non-cancerous). The remedy is very simple: give up caffeine drinks.

Hormone Effects

Our relationship with food is an uneasy one. What we eat can markedly affect our hormones. Some foods (such as soya) are known to have an estrogen-mimicking effect. Estrogen overload, as it's called, could be a marked contributor to any pain syndrome, but especially to headache, dysmenorrhea, breast discomfort, and endometriosis.

Other foods can block hormones; for example, cruciferous vegetables (cabbage, kale, broccoli, etc.) may interfere with thyroid metabolism and can lead to goiter or swelling of the thyroid gland. The technical term is a *goitrogen*.

There are still other ways in which foods can potentially cause inflammatory problems and therefore pain.

My main message is simply this: **foods can and do hurt but it's different for everyone and it is not possible to generalize which are "safe" foods and which are not.** Just figure out what's right for you and ignore everyone else's propaganda about what worked *for them*.

Could You Be Suffering from Food Allergy or Intolerance?

The big discovery in this field was that people can be highly allergic to, or intolerant of, foods and yet not be aware of it. We call it the "hidden allergy" effect. So how could you know if it was affecting you and causing or contributing to your pain?

The first thing to say is try out the program anyway. You never know till you try. Besides there are plenty of other problems that might respond well and make it more than worth the effort. For example, lack of energy or "wooly brain syndrome" are conditions that often respond very well to eliminating suspect foods.

But there are symptoms that might suggest or make it highly likely you have an allergy to one or more foods. These include the following:

- Bloating and flatulence
- Food binges
- Food cravings
- Overweight, underweight, or wildly fluctuating weight (gain a few pounds or a few inches in a day)
- Symptoms actually come on while eating
- Symptoms after food (falling asleep, chills, sudden rapid heartbeat)
- Feeling unwell without food (food addiction)
- Feeling tired, crabby or very lethargic on waking (usually because food withdrawal symptoms, as in addiction)

> Maybe that last one seems strange to you? Doesn't everybody wake up feeling bad first thing in the morning? No. It's common—but that doesn't make it normal.
>
> It has to do with the addiction basis of many food allergies and the effect of withdrawal symptoms. Think about this: by the time we wake in the morning, we may not have eaten for 10-14 hours; that's more than enough time to set up withdrawal symptoms. With breakfast, we get our first "fix" of wheat, sugar, caffeine, or whatever, and the symptoms start to clear right away.
>
> You don't believe me? Wait until you have followed the instructions in this section and you'll see the truth of what I say. It's one of the biggest surprises that comes along for many: leaping out of bed first thing in the morning, bounding with energy, bright-eyed, clear headed and in a rush to get the day's work done. Really, I'm not kidding!

The Secret of Food Allergy Test Dieting

The secret of successful identification of food allergies is to give up sufficient foods to be able to feel well, then to re-introduce these foods one at a time, so that detecting a reaction is relatively easy. We call this elimination and challenge dieting.

It rarely works to give up just one food at a time because anyone who is ill is almost certain to have more than one allergy. If it was simply one major allergen, the person would have spotted it eventually, as indeed some lucky people do. My good friend Dr Doris Rapp coined an instructive phrase: the "eight nails in the shoe trap." She points out that if you have eight nails sticking out in your shoe, and then pull *just one* of these nails, you will still limp—because of the other seven nails. It can be the same with multiple allergies. You have to work at it just that little bit harder.

Make no mistake, an elimination diet can be tough; it needs to be comprehensive, otherwise you may not get the breakthrough you are seeking (there is always unlimited amounts to eat though, you don't ever need to feel hungry).

Just bear in mind that I am talking only of a trial diet, a short-term experimental procedure. You do not need to stay on a tough diet long-term; indeed you are specifically cautioned not to do so, otherwise you run into problems caused by inadequate nutritional sources. The purpose of the strict diet is to isolate the culprits. Once you know these, you can add all the other foods back to your diet.

Then you shift into a maintenance diet, solely avoiding these offending foods, something you stay on for months or years. Almost anyone who feels much better by avoiding one or two foods has the will power to continue; the rewards are high!

Three-Tiered Plan

As I said, you may need some more in-depth help from my book Diet Wise or the Diet Wise Academy

But for this book on pain, in order to help you understand better how things work, I have prepared a three-tiered dieting system, from which you can choose the most appropriate approach for you or your family. In following the instructions it is vital that in all cases you also avoid manufactured foods. This is not because food additives are a common problem (they are surprisingly uncommon, in fact) but because manufactured foods contain numerous foodstuffs that are hidden and disguised, such as corn starch, wheat, sugar, egg and other notable allergens.

Never trust labels; food manufacturers lie blatantly, to disguise the bad things they do to adulterate what you may be eating. Stay away from food in cans, jars, bottles and packets and you'll be OK; just eat only fresh whole versions of the foods allowed.

Otherwise, it may cost you the results you are looking for.

Special note: people often ask me about using organic foods in an elimination diet. The answer is YES, *it is always better to eat organic, if you can*. But that may not be easy and it is not really necessary. Almost everyone will feel better by eating ordinary commercial food supplies, providing they are fresh. For more explicit advice on how to eat organic, consult my other writings.

Now, let's start with the easiest level diet as an entry.

An Easy Elimination Diet (14-21 Days)

It is logical to start by eliminating only the common likely food allergies. This leaves plenty of foods to eat and you should not find this diet too onerous. It is especially suitable for a child and consists basically of fresh meat, fish, fruit, and vegetables, with juice and water to drink. We call it the Paleo-, "Stone-Age" or "Caveman" diet.

FOODS YOU ARE ALLOWED TO EAT:

- Any meat (not processed or smoked)
- Any vegetables (fresh or frozen, not canned)
- Any fruit, except the citrus family (lemon, etc.)
- Any fish (not processed or smoked)
- Quinoa (grain substitute)
- All fresh unsweetened fruit juices, except citrus
- Herb teas (careful: some contain citrus peel)
- Spring water, preferably bottled in glass
- Fresh whole herbs
- Salt and pepper to taste

FOODS YOU ARE NOT ALLOWED TO EAT:

- No stimulant drinks – no tea, coffee, alcohol
- No sugar, honey, additives, or sweeteners
- No grains: absolutely no wheat, corn, rye, rice, barley, oats or millet. That means no bread, cakes, muffins, biscuits, granola, pastry, flour, or farina
- No milk or dairy produce: no skimmed milk, cream, butter, margarines or spreads, not even goat's milk
- NO MANUFACTURED FOOD: nothing from cans, packets, bottles, or jars. If somebody labeled it, they likely added to it.

Here are some important points to keep in mind:

It is vital to understand that you must not cheat on this or any other exclusion diet. This is not a slimming diet, where you can sneak a piece of chocolate cake and still lose weight. Remember that it takes several days for food to clear your bowel and eating it as little as twice a week will prevent you clearing it from your system. If you do slip up, you will need to extend the avoidance period for several more days.

Don't Forget about Addictions

It is quite likely that you will get withdrawal symptoms during the first few days. This is good news because it means you have given up something important. Usually the effects are mild and amount to nothing more than feeling irritable, tired, or perhaps having a headache, but be warned: It could put you in bed for a couple of days. I have seen wheat "cold turkey" that was just as grim as narcotics.

Please also note that it is possible to be allergic even to the allowed foods; they are chosen simply because reaction to them is less common. If you are in this minority, you might even feel worse on this diet, but at least it proves you have a food allergy. In that case, try also eliminating the foods you are eating more of (potato is a common offender) and see if you then begin to improve If not, you should switch to the Eight Foods Diet, or a half-fast, as described below.

While on the elimination diet, try to avoid hanging on to a few favorite foods and eating only those. You must eat with variety, otherwise you risk sensitizing yourself to the foods that you are eating repetitively.

Don't worry about special recipes or substitutions at this stage. By the time you have fried, baked, steamed, and grilled everything once, the two weeks will almost have passed! If, in the long term, it transpires that you need to keep off a food, then you can begin searching for an alternative.

Patients usually ask: *What about my vitamin and mineral supplements while on an elimination diet, do I need to take those?* The answer is NO. Most vitamin and mineral tablets contain hidden food ingredients, such as corn starch. Even those that say "allergy-free" formulas are misleading. They may not be made up with common allergens, such as wheat, corn, or soya derivatives; but, nevertheless, vegetable ingredients are present, such as rice polishings and potato starch. To call these allergy "safe," or even hypoallergenic, is dishonest in my view.

Don't take the risk, you won't come to any harm without supplements for a short period. Restart them when you have figured out your bandit foods!

A Word about Drugs

It is likely that you are taking pain medications, of course. Just be aware that allergies to medications are not rare and may now be contributing to the problem, rather than relieving it.

The only way to find out is to discontinue medications which are non-vital, at least for the trial period. However, certain drugs should not be stopped, such as anti-epileptics, some cardiac drugs (digoxin), insulin, and thyroxin. Some medications, such as cortisone derivatives, need to be phased out gradually.

To be certain, it is better to discuss the implications with your doctor and ask his or her advice on stopping your treatment. Don't be put off by the high-handedness which some doctors, sadly, are prone to when their prescriptions are questioned. You are entitled to know the effect of any drug you are taking and also precisely *why* you are taking it, and it may be that your doctor will not even understand the workings and side effects of drugs being used.

The key question that you want answered is, *'Will I come to harm if I stop this drug?'* Nine times out of ten the answer is, *'No'.*

Don't forget, tobacco is a drug. You *must* stop smoking if you are serious about getting well.

How Did You Get On?

If you felt a whole lot better, skip to the section below on food **challenge testing**.

DO NOT, simply because you do not improve or feel any different, make the erroneous assumption that you could not then be allergic to milk, wheat, or other banned foods. Remember the eight nails in the shoe trap? This would be a serious mistake that could bar your road to recovery. You might like to try an alternative exclusion diet, such as the nut- and pip-free or latex foods diet.

You can, in any case, carry out useful challenge tests, taking a careful note of what happens when you re-introduce a food. Careful! You do not want to hammer a pointed nail back in that shoe!

The Eight Foods Diet (7-14 Days)

Not as severe as a fast but tougher than the previous regime, is what can be called the "Few Foods Diet"; I prefer to use an eight-food plan. Obviously, it is more likely to succeed than the previous exclusion, since you are giving up more foods. Any determined adult could cope with it, but on no account should you subject a child to this diet without his or her full and voluntary cooperation. It could produce a severe emotional trauma otherwise (factually, there is rarely a problem—most children don't want to be ill and will assist you, providing they understand what you are trying to do.)

The basic idea is to produce one or two relatively safe foods for each different category we eat. Everyday foods are avoided, since these include the common allergens. Thus we would choose fruits such as mango and papaya, not apple and banana; flesh such as duck and rabbit, not beef and pork. The diet below contains my suggestions. You can vary it somewhat according to what is available to you locally.

Meat, protein	rabbit	ostrich or quail
Fruit	mango	kiwi fruit
Vegetables	spinach	sun artichoke
Starch	buckwheat	quinoa

In addition to the stipulated foods, you are allowed salt to taste but not pepper, spring water but not herb teas or juices. Even herbs and pepper must be challenged correctly on introduction. Note that neither of the starch foods is in the grains family.

The main problem with such a restricted plan is boredom. However, there is enough variety for adequate nourishment over the suggested period of five to seven days, providing you eat a balance of all eight foods. Exotic fruits can be expensive, but you won't need to eat them for long and, in any case, few people would deny that feeling well is worth any expense.

The chances are that, on a diet like this, you will feel well within 5 days, but for some conditions, such as long-standing arthritis, you will need to allow a little longer. Be prepared to go a full 10 days before deciding that it isn't working.

The Half-Fast (4-5 days)

Although a fast is the ultimate approach in tracking down hidden food allergies, I don't recommend it lightly. It is quick, inexpensive, and an absolute yes-no statement on whether your illness really is caused by food allergy.

If you stop eating altogether and your symptoms persist, then it isn't likely to be food allergy or intolerance!

The fast itself is simple enough - just don't eat for four or five days. You *must* stop smoking. Drink only bottled spring water. The whole point is to empty your bowels entirely of foodstuffs. Thus, if you have any tendency to constipation, take Epsom salts to begin with. If in doubt try an enema! Otherwise the effort may be wasted.

It may help to do what I call a grape-day step-down. This means eating grapes only for a day, as an easy step towards fasting.

A compromise with the severity of a fast is what I call a "half fast"; you eat a couple of foods that are unlikely to cause a problem. Classically, we choose lamb and pears (there is nothing to stop you picking ostrich and cantaloupe!) Fry the lamb and use the rendered fat to cook slices of pear. It's really a no-brainer.

Although it can be tough at first, by the morning of the fifth day, you can expect to feel wonderful! That's why fasting is popular as a religious exercise and why sometimes people with a severe attack of gastro-enteritis, who expel almost all the food content of the bowel by diarrhea and vomiting, are suddenly "cured" of some other health condition.

The real problem is that sometimes it can then be difficult to get back on to any safe foods. Everything is unmasked at once and the patient seems to react to everything he or she tries to eat. This can cause great distress.

Undertake a fast only if you are very determined or you still suspect food allergy and the other two approaches have failed.

Fasting is emphatically not suitable for certain categories of patient:

- Pregnant women
- Children
- Diabetics
- Epileptics
- Anyone seriously weakened or debilitated by chronic illness
- Anyone who has been subject to severe emotional disturbance (especially those prone to violent outbursts, or those who have tried to commit suicide)

Food Challenge Testing

As soon as you feel well on one of these exclusion regimes, you can begin testing, although you must not do so before the four-day unmasking period has elapsed. Allow longer if you have been constipated.

Of course, you may never improve on an elimination diet. The problem may be something else, not a food. In that case, when three weeks (maximum) have elapsed on the simple elimination diet, two weeks on the Eight Foods Diet, or seven days on a fast, then you must begin re-introducing foods.

This is vital. It is not enough to feel well on a very restricted diet; we want to know *why?* What are the culprits? These are the foods you must avoid long-term, not all those which are banned at the beginning.

Even if you don't feel well, as already pointed out, this does not prove you have no allergies amongst the foods you gave up. Test the foods as you re-introduce them, anyway - you may be in for a surprise.

My recommended procedure is as follows, except for those coming off a fast:

- Eat a substantial helping of the food, preferably on its own for the first exposure. Lunch is the ideal meal for this.

- Choose only whole, single foods, not mixtures and recipes. Try to get supplies that have not been chemically treated in any way.

- Wait several hours to see if there is an immediate reaction, and if not, eat some more of the along with a typical ordinary evening meal.

- You may eat a third, or fourth, portion if you want, to be sure.

- Take your resting pulse (sit still for two minutes) before, and several times during the first 90 minutes alter the first exposure to the food. A rise of 10 or more beats in the RESTING pulse is a fairly reliable sign of an allergy. However, no change in the pulse does **not** mean the food is safe, unless symptoms are absent also.

- If you do experience an unpleasant reaction, take Epsom salts. Also, alkali salts (a mixture of two parts sodium bicarbonate to one part potassium bicarbonate: one teaspoonful in a few ounces of lukewarm water) should help. Discontinue further tests until symptoms have abated once more. This is very important, as you cannot properly test when symptoms are already present; you are looking for foods that trigger symptoms.

Using the above approach, you should be able to reliably test one food a day, minimum. Go rapidly if all is well, because the longer you stay off a food, the more the allergy (if there is one) will tend to die down and you may miss it.

Occasionally, patients experience a "build-up" that causes confusion and sometimes failure. Suspect this if you felt better on an exclusion diet, but you gradually became ill again when re-introducing foods and can't really say why. Perhaps there were no noticeable reactions.

In that case, eliminate all the foods you have re-introduced until your symptoms clear again, then re-introduce them more slowly. This time, eat the foods steadily, several times a day, for three to four days before making up your mind. It is unlikely that one will slip the net with this approach.

Once you have accepted a food as safe, of course you must then stop eating it so frequently, otherwise it may become an allergy. Eat it once a day at most - only every four days when you have enough "safe" foods to accomplish this.

Key Points: It's important to understand that an eating test is value-less, unless you have strictly avoided the food for at least five days. Sometimes even food families cross-react, keeping each other masked, and you have to avoid the entire botanical family to get a result. Food families are beyond the scope of this book on pain.

It's not a valid test unless you eat sufficient of the food to trigger a reaction: a half liter (pint) of milk; three or four eggs; a bowlful of oatmeal; and so on.

Don't wait too long before challenge testing; the reaction might die down so that you miss it—but as soon as you start eating the food regularly, the pain will flare up again.

Special Instructions for Those
Coming off a Fast or Half-Fast

Begin only with exotic foods that you don't normally eat; *do not be tempted to grab for that coffee or cake!* The last thing you want to happen is to get a reaction when beginning to re-introduce foods – it will mean you cannot carry on adding foods until the symptoms settle down once again.

Instead, for the first few days, you want to build up a minimum range of 'safe' foods that you can fall back on. Papaya, rabbit, artichoke, and turkey, are the kind of thing to aim for - do the best you can with what is available, according to your resources.

The other important point is that you cannot afford the luxury of bringing in one new food a day: you need to go faster than this. When avoided even for as little as two weeks, a typical food allergy can die down and you may miss the proof of allergy you are looking for.

It is possible to test two or even three foods a day when coming off a fast. Pay particular attention to the pulse rate before and after each test meal and keep notes. It is important to grasp that some symptom, even if not very striking, usually occurs within the first 60 minutes of eating a food. You need to be alert to this, or you will miss items and fail to improve without understanding why.

If the worst happens and you are ill by the end of the day and can't say why, condemn all that day's new foods.

The build-up of foods is cumulative: that is, you start with Food A. If it is OK then the next meal is Food A + Food B, then A + B + C and so on.

An example table of foods tests might be:

Days 1-4	No food	
Day 5	Breakfast	Poached Salmon
	Lunch	Mango (Plus Salmon)
	Dinner	Steamed Spinach (Plus Salmon And Mango)
		No Grape On Day 5 If You Used A Grape-Day Step-Down
Day 6	Breakfast	Baked Pheasant, Quail Or Partridge, Plus Salmon, Mango And Spinach All Day, If You Desire.
	Lunch	Kiwi Fruit (Plus Any Of The Above)
	Dinner	Steamed Marrow Or Zucchini (Courgette)
Day 7	Breakfast	Lamb Chop (Plus Any Of The Above)
	Lunch	Baked Potato (Do Not Eat The Skin)
	Dinner	Banana

All safe foods are kept up after an allergic reaction. Therefore, if Food F causes a reaction, while you are waiting for it to clear up, you can go on eating foods A-E until symptoms clear.

Within a few days, you should have plenty to eat, albeit it will be monotonous. From then on, you can proceed as for those on elimination diets if you wish.

ALKALI SALTS THERAPY
In 1949, Detroit surgeon Harry G. Clark formulated a hypothesis concerning allergic reactions. He reasoned that since the end-products of digestion were acids and since the allergic inflammation process accelerated intracellular breakdown, it must be bringing about an acidic state.

Theoretically then, therapy with bicarbonate salts of sodium and potassium might be helpful in treating an acute allergic reaction. On this basis they were tried and found to be extremely beneficial. The earlier they are administered the better – after the first 24 hours they may tend to make things worse.

A mixture of two parts sodium bicarbonate to one part potassium bicarbonate is normally recommended. These can be mixed in advance and, indeed, a number of proprietary products are now available with these two salts. Malic acid may be added, merely as a flavor enhancer (otherwise the taste is rather bitter).

The usual dose is a heaped teaspoon in half a tumbler of water. This can be repeated two or three times a day but should not be used excessively, as this can be dangerous.

Also, don't forget that it makes good sense to take Epsom salts or some other simple vegetable purge (such as Senokot) if you have swallowed something that has caused a severe reaction. The faster it is cleared from the body, the better.

Your Personal Exclusion Program

Whichever exclusion program you chose, once you have carried out the challenge tests, you will have a list of items of which you are intolerant and which cause you pain or other symptoms. You must now avoid these if you are serious about your health. You have, in effect, designed your own personal diet plan for health. Use it as something you return to in times of trouble or stress, a safe platform.

There should be no rush to try and re-introduce any of these items, if at all. Design your living and eating plan without them, long-term; eat substitutes instead of battling with bandit foods.

However, the good news is that inflammatory reactions do tend to settle down over time. If you develop and practice a safer, intelligent ecological lifestyle, you may have surprisingly little further trouble. You may feel better than you have felt in years. Many patients feel and act younger, so much so that friends and relatives often comment. I noticed this over 30 years ago and that is one of the reasons I now find myself part of the anti-aging movement.

Substitutes

If you find yourself reacting to a food, you may need to seek out a substitute.

Some substitute foods are well known. If cow's milk has to be avoided, goat's milk or sheep's milk products *may* be suitable, but do test them first. Contrary to myth, goat's milk has no medicinal properties. It gets people well by getting them off cow's milk, the real cause of trouble. In fact, goat's milk is arguably a health hazard, since in some countries it isn't regulated or tested for tuberculosis and brucellosis.

Evaporated milk can be tolerated by some dairy-allergics. Heating milk changes its chemical nature and this may be enough to render it safe – but do test first, don't just make assumptions.

If wheat is a problem, try flours made from rye, barley, rice, or millet. It you find that all the grains give you problems, there are still non-cereal flours such as buckwheat (in the rhubarb family), soya, pea, potato, sago, and chestnut flours. Quinoa, a South American plant, is showing considerable promise as a grain substitute for allergics.

Eggs (to bind food) can be substituted by gram flour. There are also commercially available egg substitutes.

Finally, if you recover on an exclusion diet but can't seem to hold on to your gains, you may be developing new allergies quickly. Safe foods are breaking down and becoming reactive. The best answer to this problem is a **rotation diet** (see below).

Food Diary

It is a good idea to keep a food diary during your experiments with food. Write down everything you eat at each meal, or between meals, and also mark in any symptoms that you experience, with the time of onset in relation to meals. It is often possible to spot a pattern that recurs time and time again but which is not evident when relying only on short-term memory.

Warning: a food diary does tend to make you very conscious of food, which is probably a good thing in the short term. However, taking the long view, try to avoid becoming introverted or obsessive about your feelings and symptoms. Many allergy patients become so consumed by anxiety about what they are eating that they cannot eat or socialize normally.

Food allergy investigations, as described here, are merely a tool, not an end, and should not become a way of life, otherwise family and friends will feel excluded and that, in turn, leads to rejection.

Eating can become a psychological burden on the patient and an intolerable nuisance to family and friends, if you go too far. True health does not mean isolation from society, it means full social wellbeing included in the deal.

Key point: The food diary is merely a tool and should be discontinued as soon as practicable.

Alternative Eating Options

If the simple exclusion diet has not worked, you might like to consider alternative eliminations.

For example, you could try following a meat-free diet. Some people do feel better as vegetarians, certainly; but probably more feel ill because of the high incidence of grain and dairy allergies, as grains and dairy products are staple foods for vegetarians.

Organic Food

Some people are so highly sensitive to xenobiotic chemicals that he or she should can only be well by eating "organic." For the rest of us, it is a canon of wisdom and we must try to incorporate as much organic food in our diet as possible. Just don't be naïve and believe that every foodstuff labeled organic truly is. You need to do your homework.

It is easier nowadays to follow such an eating regime than formerly. Try it if you have reason to suspect you may be reacting to chemicals but don't go overboard; many people are convinced that pesticides on food make the mill but fail to detect them when challenged double-blind.

Organic food suppliers belong to various bodies to help them promote themselves and their ideas. Try to make contact with these organizations and find out about your local suppliers. Your local health food shop should also be able to help find locally-grown supplies.

Nut- and Pip-Free Diet

A very useful exclusion diet is the nut- and pip-free diet. This is a wide group of foods and includes a number of common allergens. Some members of this group can come as a surprise: for example, coffee is a nut.

It is an ambitious diet and it is recommended that you don't go on it until you have established a number of alternative safe foods, such as rice, rye, millet, or quinoa. Otherwise you may find yourself with very little to eat.

The following foods must be strictly avoided:

- Tomatoes, sauce, purees
- Apples, pears, plums, damsons, cherries, apricots, peaches
- Strawberries, raspberries, gooseberries, blackcurrants
- Oranges, lemons, other citrus fruits, marmalade and all fruit juices, squash, fruit-flavored drinks
- All varieties of fizzy drinks, including cola
- Jellies, instant puddings
- Chocolate, cocoa, coffee, and coffee "creamers"
- Grapes, sultanas, raisins, currants, prunes, figs, dates
- Nuts, coconut, marzipan, macaroons
- Peas, beans, lentils, soya, peanuts
- Melon, cucumber, marrow
- Spices, pepper, mustard, curry
- Cooking oils of all kinds and soft margarines
- All herbs (including mint)
- Bananas, pineapple

The Latex Foods Diet

Rubber comes from a tree and it has several botanical relatives. Latex is a common allergy; cross-reaction with these latex-lookalike foods is quite possible.

These foods are high in latex content:

- Avocado, banana, chestnut, kiwi
- These are moderate:
- Apple, carrot, celery, melons, papaya, potato, tomato

These are low in latex content or the content may simply be unknown. Therefore it would be safer to include them in the exclusion:

Apricot, cherry, citrus fruits, fig, grape, lychee, mango, nectarine, passion fruit, peach, pear, persimmon, pineapple, strawberry, buckwheat, rye, wheat, coconut, hazelnut, walnut, castor bean, chickpea, peanut, soybean, dill, oregano, sage, peppers (cayenne, sweet/bell pepper), shellfish, sunflower seed

Children

Children these days seem to have more problems than their forebears. Some have speculated that extensive vaccination programs, overwhelming the immune system, may have led to this unhappy state of affairs.

Others point to the poor nature of modern foods, vitiated of nutrients and with xenobiotic additives, which are not natural and therefore the body cannot detox safely. These, too, can hurt the immune system. It's a complex development but one which it is important we solve.

Children really need their food, to grow at the proper rate. Consider the size of a newborn infant in relation to that of an adult and you will see at once the wisdom in the old adage, "You are what you eat."

Whatever dietary experiments are undertaken with children, it is vital to see they get adequate substitutes. Milk is a problem food. It is by far the most common allergen in children. The important ingredient in milk, I believe, is not really calcium but vitamin D. Fish oils are a good alternative source. Iodine is also vital to prevent stunting and poor mental development. Since most of our supply comes from milk, alternative provision needs to be made for this element also. Kelp or iodized salt should suffice but extra iodine is always a good idea. Keep in mind that bread and other flour products often contain bromine, which displaces iodine and so easily causes a deficiency.

If you are faced with complex or long-term eliminations for your child, it is important to weigh him or her regularly (at least once a week) and keep a record of growth. Body size can be compared with charts showing average ranges for males and female youngsters and also percentiles for those who are clearly above or below average, showing how fast they should be gaining weight.

If weight gain is affected, you must get help or discontinue what you are doing. Almost no condition (the possible exception being retarded mental growth occurring because of a food allergy) is worth stunting your child's growth. It is better to defer treatment until the child is older.

Remember that withdrawal symptoms can be experienced by children, too. Be very tolerant for the first few days. He or she may crave favorite foods: just say "No" firmly and offer an alternative, Eventually, hunger will be on your side.

It's remarkable to watch how a youngster who is a faddy eater (a reliable sign of food allergy) suddenly finds his or her appetite and begins to eat heartily.

Controlling Your Food Allergies – How to Stay Well

Right, you've battled your way through to the point where you are once again reasonably pain-free and can enjoy life without endless disheartening symptoms. If you do break the rules and suffer, at least you now understand why and the bafflement is gone. How do you proceed from this point? Is it going to be a nightmare of caution and restriction for the rest of your life, no freedom, no real recovery?

The good news is NO. Almost all allergy problems will settle down and even disappear, given proper control and patience. It may take months or even years, but it is very achievable. Partly this is said in the knowledge of the way that homotoxicology (section 8) can help overcome your tendency to allergy and overload. I call sometimes call it *deep tissue cleansing* because it works deep down in the body's matrix and interstitial fluid.

Medical science ignores this critical body compartment as if it were just an afterthought of Nature, but I am quite convinced of the scientific validity of Professor Alfred Pischinger's view that it is the matrix that supports and detoxes the cells and it is therefore vitally important to keep it healthy.

The key principle involved in making a full recovery, as always, is total **body load**. Any means of reducing your health burdens will help reduce your reactivity to allergens. It's common sense! If you can bring the body load down to the point where your defenses can cope, then you will feel OK.

The most important Scott-Mumby maxim of all, based on decades of experience: **You don't need zero allergies to get zero symptoms.**

All you have to do is bring the allergy load down to within tolerable threshold limits.

Alcohol

Ethyl alcohol (ethanol) is consumed in vast quantities all over the world, indicating just how pleasurable most people find mild degrees of intoxication. There is little doubt that a meal without wine doesn't have the same warm glow that is so important to easing social tensions. The problem comes when this goes too far; excessive intake impairs your health.

Short-term side effects of drinking, such as hangover, are said to depend on "impurities," particularly the presence of other alcohols such as isoamyl alcohol, which are known as congeners. Brandy contains the highest percentage of congeners and this gives it its rich aromatic smell – enhanced by gently warming, which increases vaporization of these secondary alcohols.

For years I have been teaching that allergic reactions to foodstuffs contained in intoxicating drinks such as yeast, wheat, corn, sugar, and other ingredients are also a major cause of the negative after-effects of drinking. For example, most vodkas today are made from grains, not from potato. All alcoholic drinks are made with yeast, which will not suit someone allergic to molds and yeasts.

THE WHISKY-WHEAT TEST

I surprise people a lot when I say that, to me, bread and whisky is the same stuff! It's just wheat (or other grains) and yeast, mainly. One of the tests we used to do—it's a bit cruel but sometimes makes an important point—is have the wheat-allergic patient avoid all wheat for five days and then down a double scotch.

The pain and stiffness that results can literally put the person in bed for a few days. Just know it's a *wheat reaction*, not "alcohol."

The late, great, Theron "Ted" Randolph once described alcoholic drinks as "jet-propelled food allergy." Randolph produced a table of likely food ingredients in alcoholic drinks, which I have reproduced (with permission) many times since. Use it as a guide, to remain well while you enjoy your tipple.

However, it must be said that alcoholic drinks are largely bad news for allergics and it may be a lost cause, trying to find one you can enjoy, without it making you ill. Remember, your liver is compromised while having to detox alcohol and so cannot easily cope with other toxins at the same time. It overloads detox pathways and so reduces threshold tolerance.

While I'm on with the subject of whisky, let me tell you a story that should help bring you on board with this food-and-pain thing: it concerns a patient who had headaches almost every night, after he drank a scotch. This is a no-brainer, you would think! But actually, the food that was causing the trouble was peanuts! Every time he took a scotch he would also grab a handful of peanuts and I found that was what was really inflammatory. Stopping the whisky didn't help but stopping the peanuts cleared up the headaches for good.

Impurities

All alcoholic beverages contain yeast by definition. Also, there are many potential "additives," including sulphites and other antiseptics, letting down agents in wine such as ethylene glycol (anti-freeze), asbestos, clay, seaweed, polyvinylpyrrolidine, citric acid, tannic acid, fumaric acid, sorbates, arsenic, and monosodium glutamate. This doesn't mean all drinks include these substances, of course, simply that they may.

The point is these ingredients are potentially highly inflammatory and likely to trigger pain. You need to be careful. Remember, this is only a guide; individual products vary greatly. This is meant to help you to know what to look for.

Certain general observations will also help you make the right choice. Beers and stouts are the worst tolerated of all. Dry cider and dry white wine (including champagne), without contaminants, are the best tolerated. Red wine is usually disastrous since it may contain up to a hundred times the amount of histamine found in similar white wines. Spirits are surprisingly well taken, but people vary.

Experiment for yourself and be honest about what you find and the limitations this imposes on you.

FAQS
(FREQUENTLY ASKED QUESTIONS)

Most websites have a section called "FAQs," which stands for "frequently asked questions." Here are some FAQs on the problems of long-term management of inflammatory foods:

HOW LONG MUST I AVOID A FOOD?

This is one of the most common question asked. It's like asking, "How long is a piece of string?" To give some guidance, it may be said that major allergens should be avoided for 6 to 12 months and then tried again, using the challenge test procedure given above. If the food still causes a pain flare up or other unpleasant symptoms, wait a further 12 to 24 months before trying again. If it is still a problem, consider this a fixed allergy and keep off it.

Beware of sneaking a food back into your diet by taking tiny amounts at first, so you don't react, and then gradually increasing the quantity. This kind of self-deception will only land you back where you started – sick.

WHAT HAPPENS IF I DO EAT SOMETHING I SHOULDN'T AND I AM ILL AGAIN?

Don't panic. To help symptoms clear more rapidly, take the alkali salts mixture (below). If you don't feel much better within a few hours, take Epsom salts (magnesium sulphate) as a laxative and purge that food from your body as soon as possible. One or two heaped teaspoonfuls in half a tumbler of warm water is usually sufficient; repeat every 6-12 hours until you do evacuate.

IT WON'T DO ANY HARM IF I EAT JUST A LITTLE OF AN ALLERGY FOOD NOW AND AGAIN, SURELY?

Probably not. If your body load is comfortable, you will probably get away with, though understand you remain *highly sensitive* to an allergy food for the first few weeks after avoiding it (which is something we rely on to make challenge tests work). Do not do this often and don't cheat again if the food does trigger pain. A sore cannot heal if you keep scratching it.

I FELT GOOD AT FIRST BUT I GRADUALLY BECAME UNWELL AGAIN, DESPITE STRICTLY AVOIDING THE FOODS I SHOULDN'T. WHY IS THIS?

This almost certainly means that you have developed a new allergy among your "safe foods." This can be a troublesome problem for some individuals, where repetitive eating of a food creates new sensitivities, due to the continued exposure to the food.

In this case you will need to rotate your foods. It's too complicated to go into the full procedure here, but for your understanding, please review these important points:

Until the late twentieth century, most citizens ate off the land. There was little refrigeration and people simply ate what was available to them. Nature had her own cycles and food changed endlessly through the seasons. Foods were very varied and rotated, simply because of what was available at the time. This was a very natural way to avoid the "build-ups" that often trigger a bandit food. Now we can buy almost any food every single day of the year at the local supermarket and as a result our eating is very repetitive. It's a health hazard that most scientists and doctors are completely oblivious to.

Your answer, as a food victim, is to take charge yourself. Make a conscious effort to avoid the same foods day after day. Study food families and learn to vary the content of your diet. This can be pretty casual for some but, if your allergy problem has been severe, you will need to work out a formal planned diet scheme that we call a rotation diet (please note this has nothing to do with the rotation slimming diet that was popular in the 80s).

As I said, *Diet Wise* and its video classroom academy will help you, if you encounter this degree of difficulty.

The book: www.DietWiseBook.com

The Diet Wise Academy (over 50 videos): www.DietWiseAcademy.com

Part of the problem is ignorance, because most people are completely unaware of the origin of the foodstuffs they are eating; foods *appear* different and are made to look exciting but essentially they are the same. Bread, cakes, muffins, biscuits, crackers, pastry, pasta, pizza are all wheat products.

A family may believe each main dish as varied: beef today, chicken tomorrow, pasta the day after... yet all these servings may contain tomato and onion, which are highly repetitive foods.

The problem is made worse by modern food manufacturing. Foods are broken up and processed and the ingredients effectively disguised in the factory; yet there is wheat or corn in virtually everything that comes from a tin or packet. Foods as different as tinned soup, bouillon, ice cream, and instant coffee may all contain wheat or corn. Check the labels and see: these items appear as vegetable starch or hydrolyzed vegetable protein.

HAVE YOU ANY ADVICE ABOUT EATING OUT IN RESTAURANTS?
This is a potentially tricky situation, of course, especially if you react very violently to the wrong foods. It is tempting to avoid all risk and just stay at home. Nevertheless, I consider it vitally important to try and maintain as normal a lifestyle as possible. Otherwise you will develop reclusive tendencies and your friends and relatives will become alienated.

The most important advice is: Don't make assumptions. To protect yourself, you will need to ask pertinent questions of your server: does this dish contain any dairy products? hidden wheat? And so on. You will also need to feel you can depend on the answers. Some chefs are very tricky and may be offended if it is implied that *their* creation might make someone ill and, I'm sorry to say, may be tempted to lie about what they have done. Many chefs, apparently, have been to medical school and "know" that nobody could possibly be allergic to onions!

Which brings me to the second point: develop a few favorite places you can trust and use them, rather than being too adventurous.

THE EXCLUSION DIET WORKED WELL BUT ONCE I HAD TESTED AND RE-INTRODUCED ALL THE FOODS, I WENT BACK TO HAVING SYMPTOMS. WHY?
The fact that you did feel better means that for sure you did have food allergies. But you failed to detect them with your challenge testing and so allowed unsafe foods back in your diet. There is little choice but to go over the ground once again. Re-start the full exclusion diet for a few days, until symptoms re-clear and then re-test all the foods, going

more slowly. This time have maybe two days of steady eating on each new food, before you pronounce it safe.

I WAS DOING GREAT UNTIL I HAD A VIRUS. SINCE THEN ALL MY SYMPTOMS ARE BACK. CAN AN INFECTION REALLY DO THIS?
It certainly can. Your defense mechanisms, especially the immune system, are critical to health function. If your immune system goes under stress, because of bacterial or virus invader, the crisis can trigger the emergence of many allergies, old *and new*. I usually tell patients to go back on the exclusion program for a few days, until the crisis is past, then go back to the personal food plan.

It will also be very helpful to deploy homotoxicology remedies, to clear the intruder and its toxins as rapidly as possible and defend yourself more effectively against recurring infections.

EIGHT MEDICINE CABINET MUSTS

Every medicine cabinet should have certain basics, ready for when problems strike. You can have your paracetamol or aspirin; I'd rather have these:

Traumeel: tablets and ointment. Probably the best all-rounder in the entire canon of alternative healing (page 54).

Calendula cream: perfect for most skin worries, from burns and scalds, too much sun, to inflamed patches of all kinds (page 60).

Arnica tablets and powders: the finest instant bruising and injury, strains, sprains and wounds remedy there is. 30C (page 111).

Recue remedy: never let anyone feel hurt, shocked or upset, without giving Bach's Rescue remedy (page 59)

An Avazzia device: if you can afford one, be sure to learn how to use it. It's good for almost anything, from kidney stones, to injury; fractures, wounds, sprains and punctures; diabetic ulcers; migraines; toothache and beyond (page 85).

Oil of Cloves. Best first remedy for toothache. Rub raw, warmed oil of cloves into the gum (page 117).

Peppermint Oil. Great if humble indigestion and bellyache remedy (page 116).

Final Tip: grow yourself an Aloe vera plant! There is no more healing plant or better remedy in all of nature. It will heal anything from colitis to sunburn; sore throat and cystitis to headache. This cactus/succulent is proverbially easy to grow. It loves us humans and does it's very best to be helpful and accommodating! Break a bit off and rub the slippery, slimy surface onto the injured part of the body.

APPENDIX

YOUR PAIN DIARY

WHAT IS A PAIN DIARY?

A pain diary is a written record of the levels of pain you have been experiencing on a daily basis. It helps you to describe to your healthcare team how your pain has been affecting you over time.

A pain diary also records how medicines, other therapies and your activities influence your pain levels throughout the day.

WHY SHOULD I KEEP A PAIN DIARY?

A pain diary can help you and your healthcare team:

- Recognize how well pain management is working
- Learn what most influences your pain levels
- Understand what makes your pain worse and what helps to relieve your pain, including changes in your medicines or other therapies.

WHEN SHOULD I USE A PAIN DIARY?

Use your pain diary whenever you feel it's appropriate or as recommended by your doctor or pharmacist.

It may be more important in the early stages, when pain control methods are being tried. If your pain is under control you may not need to use the diary as often.

Don't be afraid to add notes. The more information you record in your pain diary, the more helpful it will be for you and your healthcare team.

HOW DO I COMPLETE A PAIN DIARY?

Record all the information that is relevant to your pain in the diary over the page. You may not need to fill out all columns each time.

Use the rating chart (below) to rate your pain. A zero (0) means no pain and a ten (10) means worst possible pain. Select the number that best describes your pain. You can use half points if you wish (eg. 7½ if it's more than 7 but less than 8).

Use the same rating scale to rate the 'relief' of your pain (select the number that indicates how your pain feels after you took action).

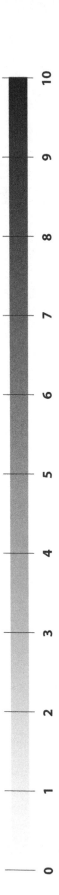

0 1 2 3 4 5 6 7 8 9 10

DATE	TIME	DESCRIBE YOUR PAIN (it's character, location, duration, etc.)	RATE YOUR PAIN (0–10)	ANYTHING MADE YOUR PAIN WORSE? (therapy, medication, herbal, etc.)	WHAT PAIN TREATMENTS WERE TRIED? (medicine or nonmedicine e.g. exercise)	RATE THE RELIEF OF YOUR PAIN – INCLUDE TIME UNTIL RELIEF (0–10)	COMMENTS (e.g. problems with medicines, how your pain affects your daily life – sleep, mood, work etc.)

PAIN SUPPORT GROUPS AND AGENCIES

ALL LINKS WERE LIVE, AS OF 22ND JUNE 2014.
Note that none of these websites are recommended or guaranteed to be friendly towards natural remedies. You will have to satisfy yourself whether the "support group" is a clever Big Pharma drug-pushing front group or not (some are).

USA Pain Support Organizations

The American Academy of Pain Management
http://www.aapainmanage.org

The American Chronic Pain Association
http://www.theacpa.org/Support-Groups

Pain Connection
http://painconnection.org/support/index.html

Geisinger Interventional Pain Center Support Groups
http://www.geisinger.org/services/pain/support.html

Trigeminal neuralgia' The Facial Pain Support group
http://www.fpa-support.org

Arthritis Foundation
http://www.arthritis.org/

Fibromyalgia Network
http://www.fmnetnews.com

The Mayday Fund
mayday@maydayfund.org
www.painandhealth.org

National Cancer Institute (NCI)
cancer.gov_staff@mail.nih.gov h
ttp://cancer.gov

National Chronic Pain Outreach Association (NCPOA)
ncpoa@cfw.com
www.chronicpain.org

National Fibromyalgia and Chronic Pain Association
www.fmcpaware.org

National Foundation for the Treatment of Pain
NFTPain@cwo.com
www.ninds.nih.gov/find_people/voluntary_orgs/volorg711.htm

National Headache Foundation
info@headaches.org
www.headaches.org

Neurofibromatosis, Inc. (NF Inc.)
info@nfinc.org
www.nfinc.org

Trigeminal Neuralgia Association
2801 SW Archer Road Suite C Gainesville, FL 32608
Tel: 352-376-9955 Fax: 352-376-8688
tnanational@tna-support.org
www.tna-support.org

National Headache Foundation
http://www.headaches.org

The Neuropathy Association
www.neuropathy.org

NIH Pain Consortium
http://painconsortium.nih.gov/index.html

Pain.com (The Dannemiller Memorial Educational Foundation)
www.pain.com

Pain Institute Leadership Council
www.medscape.com/infosite/paininstitute/article-1

PainKnowledge.org
www.painknowledge.org

Pain Management by MedicineNet.com
www.medicinenet.com/pain_management/article.htm

Partners Against Pain
www.partnersagainstpain.com

WebMD Pain Management Health Center
www.webmd.com/pain-management/default.htm

Cancer Pain Management in Children
www.childcancerpain.org/

Cancer Pain Management at the MD Anderson Cancer Center
www.mdanderson.org/topics/paincontrol/

Cleveland Clinic Anesthesiology Institute Pain Management
http://my.clevelandclinic.org/anesthesiology/pain-management

Power Over Your Pain
www.poweroveryourpain.com/sb/index.html

Stanford School of Medicine Pain Management Center
http://paincenter.stanford.edu/

Spine Universe
www.spineuniverse.com/displayarticle.php/article3336.html

UK Pain Support Resources

Pain Relief Foundation
http://www.painrelieffoundation.org.uk

Action On Pain
http://www.action-on-pain.co.uk

British Pain Society
http://www.britishpainsociety.org.uk

Chronic Pain Policy Coalition
www.policyconnect.org.uk/cppc

Pain Concern
http://painconcern.org.uk

Pain Support
http://www.painsupport.co.uk

Pain Community Centre
www.paincommunitycentre.org

Neuropathy Trust
www.neurocentre.com

Arthritis Research UK
www.arthritisresearchuk.org/arthritis-information.aspx

The Patient's Association
www.patients-association.com

Mood Juice Chronic Pain
www.moodjuice.scot.nhs.uk/chronicpain.asp

Bandolier (authoritative guide)
www.medicine.ox.ac.uk/bandolier/booth/painpag/

Australia and New Zealand
Pain Support Resources

Managing Acute Pain (authoritative pdf)
www.painaustralia.org.au/images/pain_australia/Healthcare/managingacutepain.pdf

Australian Family Physician Pain
www.racgp.org.au/afp/2013/march/mind-body-therapies/

Pain Australia (variety of downloadable pdf reports)
www.painaustralia.org.au

Chronic Pain Australia
www.chronicpainaustralia.org.au

New Zealand resources For Life
www.life.org.nz/euthanasia/euthanasiamedicalkeyissues/pain-relief/

Made in the USA
Monee, IL
07 September 2023

42295760R10144